Health is wealth

April 18, 2018
atozhealthguide.com

Life Begins at 65

Words of a Cancer Survivor

by

Matthew E. McLaren

authorHOUSE®

AuthorHouse™
1663 Liberty Drive, Suite 200
Bloomington, IN 47403
www.authorhouse.com
Phone: 1-800-839-8640

This book is a work of non-fiction. Unless otherwise noted, the author and the publisher make no explicit guarantees as to the accuracy of the information contained in this book and in some cases, names of people and places have been altered to protect their privacy.

© 2008 Matthew E. McLaren. All rights reserved.

No part of this book may be reproduced, stored in a retrieval system, or transmitted by any means without the written permission of the author.

First published by AuthorHouse   12/4/2008

ISBN: 978-1-4389-0379-8 (sc)

Printed in the United States of America
Bloomington, Indiana

This book is printed on acid-free paper.

Foreword

The words, "prostate cancer", overheard in casual conversation are enough to cause the average male to cringe. To actually be diagnosed with this condition is to many a devastating blow from which they never recover, neither emotionally nor physically. Matthew McLaren received the blow and turned it into a twofold opportunity. First, he overcame his own cancer. Secondly, he gave us detailed roadmaps so that others in the same situation can find their way out of it – or better yet, to bypass the quagmire entirely by taking simple preventative measures.

This book is "must" reading both for anyone who has prostate cancer (or wishes to prevent it) and for anyone who treats this condition (or dispenses information about it). Within these covers, Matthew has created a virtual encyclopedia of the etiology, anatomy, physiology, biochemistry and treatments of prostate cancer – written in a style that is easy to understand by lay people and thorough enough for practitioners. He interweaves science and personal experience in a delightful way.

The theme of this book is self-empowerment. Our body comes with its own innate healing power. It can cure itself of any condition – provided we give it the conditions it needs to do so, and in a timely manner. Matthew details what those conditions are. Much of the wisdom he expresses herein applies not only to prostate cancer but also to other forms of cancer and to disease in general.

Mind and body are not two but one. Many diseases are created by negative thoughts, especially those which are repetitive and deeply engrained. The surest way to create a favourable outcome for any disease is to change the conditions that created it, both physical and mental. Characteristically, people with cancer don't feel entitled to express negative feelings, including anger. They keep these negative feelings bottled up, eating away inside, so to speak. The longer one does this, the more he will feel helpless and that his situation is hopeless. Matthew points a way out of all this. Follow his lead. Don't take anything at face value. Question everything. Examine all your options. Choose the ones that feel best to you. Do this and you will be self-empowered. Hopelessness and helplessness will then be in your past, as will your cancer.

Matthew has left no stone unturned. He presents a wide range of both medical and alternative therapies from which to choose. His descriptions of each are thorough, objective and non-judgmental. The more informed you are and the more options you have, the more power you have to create the outcome you desire. "There are many paths up the mountain, but the view from the top is the same."

Read and enjoy,

- *David W. Rowland*

Acknowledgement

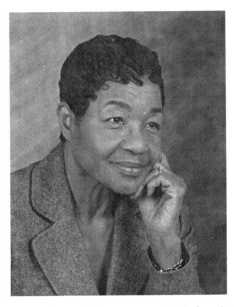

I would like to give acknowledgment to God for divine healing and wisdom, to my wife Theresa for her 44 years of continuous love and support. To my dear wife I say, 'I never thought I'd find a life partner with so much strength and compassion; a woman with such integrity and goodness in her heart…The more I know you, the deeper I appreciate and love you. It's like how I'd cherish and enjoy a rare and priceless work of art. I realize you may not be as perfect as I see you, yet in my eyes and in my heart, there's no one else on earth more genuine and precious than you, my one and only love. And there's no treasure anywhere to equal what you're worth.' Thanks also to my children Jackie, Courtney, Ken, Caphelle and their spouses for their encouragement and support, also to my church family and pastors, for 46 years of spiritual guidance. Finally, thanks to Edison Institute of Nutrition, and Dr. David Rowland for the solid foundation they provided me in Science of Nutrition. My appreciation also goes to Westbrook University for my Doctoral program in Philosophy of Nutrition.

Introduction

The purpose of this book is to identify in greater depth and fullness, my ability to withstand difficulties and setbacks in life and view them as learning experiences. The most important factors on which our characters are defined are our ability to perform and succeed in difficult and stressful conditions. Age or sickness should not dictate our ability to take immediate control of our mental, physical, spiritual, emotional, and financial destiny. Faith and belief in our true worth in this journey of life can strengthen or weaken our ability to achieve optimum health and wealth.

For Theresa and me, we truly believe that life begins at 65. At 65 I retired from The Regional Municipality of Durham Duffin Creek Incineration Plant as a shift engineer. Soon after, I began a new career as a nutrition consultant. I've always had a desire to be a Christian motivational speaker, to promote God's amazing grace of health and wealth of mind-body. Retirement has provided me with the freedom to pursue my dream. In this journey of life, age does not determine our success in accomplishing tasks enroute to our destination.. I have a special message for all seniors, cancer survivors and survivors of other illnesses. My simple message is this: Age and sickness do not have to determine where our lives end or the quality of life we live. Age is a unique and priceless treasure that can provide wisdom and knowledge which cannot be learned in university and text books. This wisdom can only be accumulated by years of experience within our environment and an intimate relationship with our Creator.

Our Creator has designed within us a mind-body that is special and unique to humans. It's true our mind-body is constantly facing attacks from foreign invaders that could cause infection, illness and disease. These 'attacks' include living microbes in the form of bacteria, fungi, parasites, and viruses; non-living toxins, such as man-made chemicals and drugs. The mind-body is fortified with a number of external and internal safeguards that prevent most dangerous invaders from entering our body and causing harm. The physical barriers are referred to as our body's front-line defence systems.

Our skin, the body's largest organ, provides physical and chemical barriers against outside environment. This organ forms a protective layer that completely surrounds the mind-body. It protects our cells, tissues, blood vessels, bones, organs and systems. When we get a cut or injury to our skin, this could provide an entrance for infective agents. Certain glands established beneath the skin activate special enzymes that help to kill the bacteria. Areas of our mind-body that are not protected by the skin are protected by other defensive measures. Mucus membranes line the respiratory system and secrete mucus that traps irritants that enters through the nose. There are other protections that prevent foreign particles from entering the lungs. Harmful microbes that escape and enter the stomach are destroyed by stomach acids.

Our brain is surrounded by a brain blood barrier that acts as a physical shield to keep out toxins and most microbes while letting in glucose, which is a source of nutrients for the brain. Other lines of defence are equipped within the mind-body. These include the nervous, endocrine and immune systems that are designed to recognize and destroy all foreign invaders that enter the mind-body. Our Creator has uniquely designed our immune system with the ability to identify and destroy antigens, and to remember the markers of the antigens it has been exposed to, so that the body can provide a better and faster immune response the next time these antigens re-enter the body.

As we grow older, these defence systems require more need for penetrative maintenance. This does not limit our ability to perform and enjoy an active lifestyle of optimum health and wellness. If our mind-body does not keep active, physically, mentally, spiritually, and emotionally, we will rust out and decay. The human body is designed and uniquely structured to last for more than one hundred years, when properly maintained. Some researchers and health care professionals have suggested that the reason we experience such degenerative diseases as cancer, heart problems and the like, is that people are living longer. This could be true for a small percentage of our society.

However, according to a recent study conducted by the American Institute for Cancer Research, one-third of all cancers are preventable through a combination of dietary changes, adequate physical activity, and maintenance of appropriate body weight. Avoiding tobacco and alcohol could prevent an additional one-third of the occurrences of cancer. The report suggested that 200,000 of the 600,000 cancer deaths in the United States each year might be prevented if these recommendation guidelines were followed.

The concept of preventing or influencing the growth of cancer has been studied since the early 1900s. In 1942 Tannenbaum described the enhanced effect a high-fat diet had on tumor growth and in animal models. In 1981 Doll and Peto reported that dietary factors may account for 35 percent of cancer deaths, and a report published by the National Academy of Science in 1982 presented convincing evidence about the relationship between dietary fat and cancer. Citizens need to be better educated about health issues. Education could reduce the cost of health care within our community.

The role of the diet in the prevention and management of prostate cancer is undergoing intensive investigation. There are multiple causes of prostate cancer involving the aging process, hereditary factors, hormonal influences, and environmental factors. Perhaps the most important environmental factors are diet and lifestyle.

Researchers have accumulated information indicating that diet and lifestyle play an important role in the prevention and management of disease. Epidemiologic, animal model, biochemical, molecular biological, and cell culture studies are being done to evaluate the effect of nutrition and dietary supplements on the development and prevention of cancer. These studies have begun to yield results that allow health care professionals, to advise patients regarding their diets. The studies should include information on emotional stressors, which multiply our problems.

The presence of prostate cancer cells is surprisingly common. Autopsy studies have shown that cancer cells can be detected within the prostate in 26 percent of men aged thirty to forty years and 38 percent of men in their fifth decade. Prostate cancer cells seem to exist either as latent cancers whose numbers expand very slowly, which is the situation in 85 percent of men, or as actively growing cancers with the ability and propensity to metastasize. Researchers say this change in behaviour from a slow-growing, latent cancer to aggressive carcinoma is not clear, but it is the subject of intense investigation.

Contents

Chapter 1: My Personal Experience with Prostate Cancer 1

Chapter 2: An Overview of Prostate 23

Chapter 3: Prostate Disorder Diagnosis and Treatment 31

Chapter 4: Treatment of Prostate Cancer: The Conventional Methods 55

Chapter 5: Living with Side Effects Caused by Conventional Treatments 67

Chapter 6: An Alternative Approach to Prevention and Treatment 81

Chapter 7: Preventative Maintenance and Management of Mind/Body: 119

Chapter 8: Conclusion 151

Glossary 173

Bibliography 181

Chapter 1:
My Personal Experience with Prostate Cancer

On July 10, 1997, I almost became a statistic. Fear, anger, and total shock sent my emotions skyrocketing. That was the day I found out I had prostate cancer. The news came after a visit to my doctor for a routine checkup. After doing a digital rectal examination (DRE), he started going through my file. A few moments later he looked up from the file and curiously asked, "What have you done about your prostate cancer?" "My what?" I blurted back, hoping I hadn't heard right. "Your prostate cancer," he repeated. I could hardly believe what I was hearing. Panic and fear took over, and then anger and frustration set in. You see, a year earlier, I had taken a prostate specific antigen test (PSA). The reading was 5.8, and I was referred to an urologist. There he did a biopsy to determine malignancy. Days, weeks, months, and a year passed and I didn't hear from either doctor, so I assumed the result was negative. After all "no news is good news," or so I thought. Just imagine the shock and frustration I felt when my doctor asked that dreaded question.

"Why wasn't I informed?" I demanded. I literally lost it. I was enraged. I could feel the physical (fight or flight) responses setting in. But reality soon struck me, irrespective of who was to be blamed; the fact was that I had cancer. I left the doctor's office in a daze. Driving home my mind wandered back to my late father, and the physical and mental anguish he suffered just before he died. He literally deteriorated to a mere skeleton. My late mother told me she prayed for him to die so that he could be relieved from his pain and suffering. I remembered my trip to the morgue. His frame was so emaciated; at first I did not recognize him, and I cried.

Remembering my mother, I initially decided not to tell my wife, but better judgment prevailed and I told her. Much to my surprise, she handled the news better than I expected. That gave me strength. I decided at the time not to take conventional treatment. I was going to change my diet and continue with my life, but things didn't work out that way. From there everything went downhill, or so I thought. That very week, my employer informed me that my job was about to become redundant. As if prostate cancer was not enough, I was now facing unemployment. A blister broke on my hand and began spreading to about the size of a quarter, and other small ones came out on my fingers. In my mind I thought the cancer was spreading. Another PSA test came back with a higher reading: 6.4. Everything seemed to be going out of control. I prayed. But that "mustard-seed" faith was lacking. The faith that brought instantaneous healing to my body many years ago when I was first diagnosed with diabetes was now inadequate. During this time my life took on new meaning. I became very contemplative and began questioning my purpose in life and its fulfillment. This led to an awakening of a deeper desire for spiritual growth and further information on the laws of health to develop physical, mental, and emotional strength.

I began reading all I could on cancer. My wife was very supportive in gathering information from various sources, including the Canadian Cancer Society. Her nursing experience provided her with added strength and support when it was needed most. After much research and consultation, I decided to proceed with surgery. The surgery was successful and I gave God thanks, because I know that even though it is the doctor who does the cutting, it is God who does the healing. I feel especially blessed because one does not just "cut out" cancer and live happily ever after.

The statistics for longevity after cancer surgery are uncertain. Cancer generally reappears if preventive measures are not taken. Today, my lifestyle is completely reformed in accordance to the natural health laws that God gave to us from the beginning, to enjoy happiness and abundant living. I am living with side effects from the surgery, but I gain strength from adversities. With my loving and caring wife by my side, I am guided by the Bible verse "All things work together for good to them that love the Lord." Knowledge, strength, and mental success are gained from experience. Because I have walked this pathway before, I can help others who may follow the same path. The physical, mental, and emotional pain has given me experience, which allows me the opportunity to leave signposts to guide others safely through this life's rugged terrain. Today I am not only physically and spiritually healthy, but I am in control of my life and have now made it my personal responsibility to take a proactive role in the fight against prostate cancer and other cancers. My quest to learn more about healthy living has provided me with incentives to train as a nutrition consultant.

My experience and training has shown me that there is a powerful healing capacity within me. This innate intelligence is working constantly to restore the balance and harmony of health and wellness. As a child of God, I now know that I have more control over my health than we have been taught. My health is my responsibility. I have the choice to determine what I put in my body and what lifestyle I live. If I give up that responsibility to a stranger, I become disempowered and de-energized. I do not see myself as a survivor; I see myself living a life of high self-esteem filled with energy and vitality. "Yesterday is but a dream and tomorrow only a vision, but today well lived, makes every yesterday a dream of happiness and every tomorrow a vision of hope" (Kalidasa - An ancient Indian poet.).

There are many health challenges, and I am conscious that life is filled with positives and negatives. I have learned to face my greatest fear with the understanding that I am not alone and that I have family and friends, but most of all I have God. Two of my powerful tools are prayer and meditation. I learned to visualize the healing power of God. Since my surgery on November 17, 1997, I have not taken any prescription drugs. I have been given prescriptions for drugs but I have never filled them, because I did not believe they were necessary. If I had ever needed them I would have taken them. You see many of us were made to believe that our health is something that only doctors and prescription drugs can influence. We are culturally programmed to expect fast cures for our ills and look to others for answers. After my surgery the urologist recommended that I take radiation treatment as a precaution against cancer cells that may have been left behind because of the enlargement of my prostate. I gracefully declined. My concern was the added stress on my body and that good cells would have been compromised and in turn weakened my immune system against pathogens.

I do believe that the majority of medical professionals are dedicated to their work and are doing a good job in the area of medicine in which they have been trained. They should be commended. However, after my first experience with surgery, I have decided to take a proactive role in decision making that involves my health. I can vividly remember an incident that took place in the recovery room after the surgery. My heart was fluctuating rapidly. I was supposed to go to the recovery room for a few minutes, but I ended up in the intensive care unit for three days under observation for heart problems. I was asked several questions about the previous condition of my heart. Several tests were conducted, and the medical staff could not come up with any answers. Everyone was getting very concerned, excluding myself because my faith and my belief in God gave me strength. It was on the third day when a student doctor suggested that they reduce the fluid I was receiving via the IV machine. After the reduction my heart went back to a normal rhythm.

My other experience was with the urologist who did the surgery. He was very devoted during my stay in the hospital and during the time I had the catheter in place. I remember when he was going to remove the catheter. He would not do it in his office. He took me over to the hospital, where he could use the endorectal MRI to see that the removal was carefully done. His remark was, "I have never lost one before so I don't want to begin now." I presumed he was referring to incontinence.

Before the surgery he had told me that all his patients regained control of their urinary functions. After the catheter was out and I gained urinary bladder control, his attitude changed, and he would not take time to answer my questions and give relevant information. I knew he was never a person with doctor-to-patient communication skills. I had never felt relaxed and comfortable talking to him. In one of our preliminary discussions before the surgery, I tried to discuss the subject of impotence. He told me he was trained to save lives and not to prevent impotence. For some men this is their life, and this subject should not have been taken lightly when a person is in their most vulnerable state of illness. This attitude could become demoralizing to a doctor-patient relationship. (One prostate cancer survivor told me that when he found out he was impotent after surgery, he went into depression for eighteen months.) His aggressive impatient attitude during my follow-up visits for the test and assessments became tense and unacceptable. The atmosphere was not conducive to mental and physical healing. I made the decision to cut off my visits. I came to the conclusion that he was not interested in me as a person. He was interested in the disease and his reputation as a successful urologist. This reminded me of Dr. Siegel's reference to the young doctors who referred to a sick little girl as "an interesting case." Dr. Bernie Siegel said in his book, *Love Medicine and Miracle*, that the experience changed his attitude toward his patients. He began to see his patient as a person and not as a label. He stated that the change was well worth it, because it broke down the barrier between him and his patients. And for the first time he began to empathize fully about what it meant to live with an illness.

A word of commendation for my family doctor is after the first incident with the biopsy report he has since taken special interest in my regular visits and is very supportive. He has a doctor-patient relationship that says, "I do care."

"Information doesn't change anyone; inspiration does." I have found my reason to live, which inspired me to higher consciousness of divine healing and to eliminate fear and guilt. Inspiration resurrects joy, contentment, serenity, and peace in knowing that sickness and trials do not come to stay; they come to pass. Physicians do not have the ultimate say about our state of health. In a very real way, we can become our own doctors. The word "doctor" is derived from the Latin word "teach." We can teach our bodies to function at their maximum efficiency, drawing from the miracle of modern medicine only when we need to augment our natural healing system. Our Creator has provided us with the capacity to think, to feel in ways that can protect us from disease, to heal us when we are sick, and to help us to attain a new level of wellness, a level far beyond the mere absence of symptoms of diseases. When I visualize his healing power, I know that each thought, feeling, and emotion stimulates the potential chemical messengers and prepares them as an army to defend against terrorist invaders of my homeland (the body's immune system).

When I focus on helping others, I do not have time to feel sorry for myself. My mind is occupied with positive emotions. Feelings of ecstasy envelope my mind and body and bring about harmonious healing and a sense of gratitude filled with joy and acceptance of my family and the people around me. The acid test of my life is to live one day at a time and enjoy each moment while it lasts. It is not how long I live that is important, it is the quality of the life I live and the influence that I have on those I come in contact with each day. The relationship that exists between the mind and body is very intimate. When one is affected, the other sympathizes. The condition of the mind affects our health to a far greater degree than many realize. Many of the diseases from which we suffer are the result of mental depression, grief, anxiety, discontent, remorse, guilt, and distrust. All tend to break down our life forces and to invite decay and death.

In October of 2002 I went to my doctor for my regular checkup. He did some blood tests. Two weeks after the tests, my doctor called me; he was concerned because my white blood counts were very low. He told me he was concerned because there was a consistent drop in the various tests over a period of time, which he suggested was not good. He requested that I come back and repeat the blood tests. I discussed the situation with my wife. I told her I was concerned, but I was not worried. I told her that we would take it to God in prayer, because I know that I can do all things through Christ, who strengthens me. We prayed, and I give thanks to God for answered prayer.

I repeated the blood tests; the doctor's secretary called and informed me that the test was OK. However, the doctor wanted me to take a bone marrow biopsy as a precaution. He made the appointment with an oncologist. I took the bone marrow test, and the result was good. Bone marrow biopsy is a procedure whereby a needle is inserted into a bone to obtain a sample of cells of the bone marrow. Bone marrow biopsy is valuable for establishing a specific diagnosis for several groups of blood diseases. These can include anemia, leukemia and lymphoma.

Our bone marrow is essential to good health. Stem cells are manufactured within the bone marrow. Other cells are produced from stem cells. Red blood cells, for example, are responsible for transporting oxygen and nutrients to tissue and organs to provide energy and life; white blood cells, on the other hand, provide security for our mind-body, and protect it from such internal and external enemies as bacteria, virus, and pathogens. Platelets clot our blood, and prevent us from bleeding to death, if we get a cut or injury.

Blood Cells
- Red blood cell
- White blood cell
- Platelets

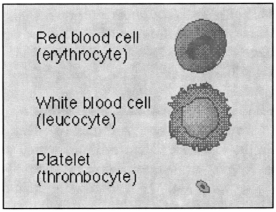

"Taken from CancerHelp UK"

Knowing the reason for these medical tests, and the positive or negative effects the result could have on our mind-body, can often create stressors that are synonymous of emotions. Such stressors are shock, fear anger, and other depressive stress symptoms. These challenges have given me strength to help others who are afflicted with prostate or other cancers. I continue to live by faith and trust in the one who heals.

On September 6, 2007, nine years four hundred and forty-four days after my surgery for prostate cancer, I was back in the same hospital with the same urologist having surgery for hydrocele. I made the decision to go with the same urologist because of his excellent skill as a surgeon and his track record for success. After the experience with this surgery, I have not changed my mind about his doctor-to-patient communication skills. If anything, I came away more impressed with the fact that he takes extra-special interest in his patients. My visit to his office for treatment for the hydrocele was eight years after I thought I would never go back to see him. After his examination of my scrotum and prostate, he looked at me and said "Someone up there is taking care of you." I can only concur: Yes, someone has been taking special care of me. Since my surgery for prostate cancer, I have not taken any radiation, chemotherapy or medication. I regularly supply my mind-body with essential high-performance fuel, as required by our Creator's manual. After all, he has designed my structure with such skill, precision, and complexity, it deserves to be taken care of. A balanced diet of wholesome natural foods; clean water, fresh air, exposure to sunlight; exercise, relaxation and proper rest are the minimal nutrients it needs. Guided by temperance, faith and trust in God's divine grace and mercy, I have been divinely blessed with a unique healing system. With the previously mentioned essentials, my mind-body continues its healing process daily.

Although hydrocele is an abnormal defect within the urinary and reproductive system, it is not a prostate problem. Many people called when I was in the hospital to find out if the cancer had returned. I assured them that my prostate was not a problem. Hydrocele is a swelling of the scrotum caused by a collection of fluid in the tunica vaginalis testis, the outermost covering of the testes. It can be removed by withdrawing (aspirate) the fluid by tapping through the outer layer of the tissue. However, hydroceles that are aspirated often reoccur. An operation that cuts away the outer layer of the tissue makes it more difficult for the hydrocele to return. Aspiration is recommended only for men who are not physically able to have surgery.

Urinary System and Organs
- Scrotum
- Testis
- Tunica Vaginalis

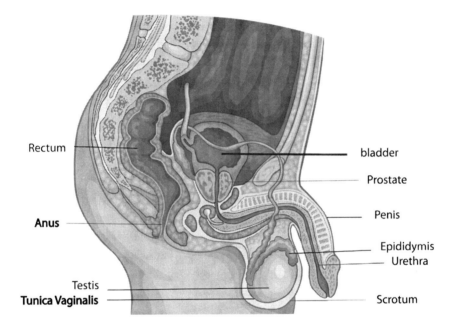

About one out of every ten infant males has a hydrocele at birth, but most hydrocele disappears within the first year of life, without treatment. When a hydrocele appears later in life, it may be caused by an injury or surgery to the scrotum or groin area. This can be due to inflammation or infection of the epididymis or testicles. Hydrocele may also occur with cancer of the testicle. This type of hydrocele mostly occurs in men over age forty. Often a hydrocele does not cause symptoms, but can become very uncomfortable.

Hydrocele is filled with fluid which will allow light to shine through it. Light will not shine through a solid mass of tissue; that may be caused by other problems, such as cancer of the testicle. For diagnosis, a doctor can shine a light behind each testicle to check for solid mass. An ultrasound may be recommended to confirm the diagnosis. I believe the cause of my hydrocele, is an ill-advised surgery I had many years ago. We should not experiment with our bodies. It is only advisable to have surgery when it is absolutely necessary. All surgeries are stressful to our mind-body, and can cause regrettable side effects.

After my surgery, I was discharged from the hospital on November 7. On November 21 - my second visit for my check-up after surgery - my scrotum was swollen to about one- and-one-half its size before the surgery. I had a problem walking. The doctor withdrew several cubic centremetres of blood, from the scrotum. It had accumulated, because of internal bleeding. He advised me to go home and lie on my back, with my legs elevated. He also recommended blood tests for my platelet and white blood count. The tests came back with a low platelet reading.

On November 23 my scrotum started passing lots of pale blood mixed with pus. It carried an offensive odor. I immediately called my wife, who is also a nurse. She was at work and she had me rushed to the hospital. The urologist on call wanted to operate immediately to clear up the infection. My wife and I did not like the idea. We suggested that he withdraw the fluid to relieve the pressure and allow my urologist to make the final decision. He withdrew approximately half a liter of pus mixed with blood from my scrotum.

The following day my urologist came to see me on the ward. He informed me that the blood test results showed that my white blood count and platelet were low. He suggested that he would continue the antibiotic, and ordered Vitamin 2K for clotting of my blood. He would also consult with the hospital hematologist before making any further decision. I was very disappointed because the swelling of my scrotum was like a mountain between my legs. It was painful and I had a temperature. My wife and I were concerned. I could not prevent my thought from going back to my experience of July 10, 1997, when I was told I had prostate cancer. Infections that require surgery leave me with unpleasant thoughts, but as usual, whenever I find myself falling prey to negative thoughts, I shift my focus to God, who provides strength and healing.

Bacteria and Virus that cause infections

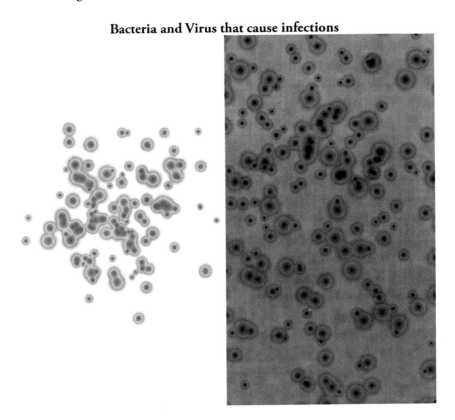

The hematologist specialist came to see me. In our discussion he assured me that there was nothing wrong with my platelet, or white blood cells (lymphocytes). He suggested that it is natural for the blood platelet and white blood count to fluctuate, because the immune system is fighting the bacteria or virus that causes the infection. He also provided me with added information. He informed me that the white blood count of Black people is normally lower than the count of some races. This is the second time I have heard this statement. I will be doing some intensive research on this topic, to be better informed and be in a position to provide relevant information.

By November 30, there was still no relief for the swelling and accompanying discomfort. I prayed earnestly for relief. The same night I experienced a miracle: my scrotum was opened by divine hands. The infected content flowed out, saturating the bed. The following day the urologist came to see me. He pointed to my Bible and suggested that "someone up there" has been taking care of me. This was the second time he had made that statement. I was very pleased with his comment, because most doctors do not give credit to God for healing. Before the scrotum became infected I had been informed by my doctor that the healing process would take about three months. It took six weeks. Doctors can diagnose and treat diseases, surgeons can wield a scalpel but only our healing system, through God's power, can do the healing. Our Creator has equipped our body with all the necessary equipment to repair damage. However, there are times when we have to request divine intervention for healing. More than 2000 years ago, Hippocrates, who is considered "the father of medicine," stated that "the natural forces within us are the true healer of disease."

In the book Ministry of Healing, E.G. White, writes, "There are thousands who can recover health if they will. The Lord does not want them to be sick. He desires them to be well and happy, and they should make up their mind to be well. Often invalids can resist disease simply by refusing to yield to ailments, and (they) settle down in a state of inactivity. Rising above their aches and pains, let them engage in useful employment suited to their strength. By such employment (of) the free use of air and sunlight, many an emaciated invalid might recover health and strength."

We need to take time to learn more about the incredible healing system within us. Our mind-body is an incredible creation. There is no man-made machine in this world that can compare to it. It is designed and crafted by the master designer who has created the universe. Although we have abused it immensely, it keeps on ticking. Many of us take better care of our cars and our homes than we do of our bodies. It is a miracle many of us are alive. I'm familiar with a man who had surgery for lung cancer. The first chance he had to leave his bed, what did he do? He went out for a smoke. Men are less likely to take special care of their health. Wives are more concerned about their husband's health. Men need to know that whenever they get sick, or whenever they die, it affects the lives of their families. I read an article where several men stated that they would rather die by prostate cancer than take treatment that could leave them impotent. I hope I can motivate men to become more proactive about their health. This is why I am giving so much information about my personal experience with surgery. Sickness is nothing to be ashamed of. Not taking action to support our body with the essential factors it needs to prevent sickness and giving it the opportunity to provide healing if we get sick, is a major problem!

I am so fascinated with the incredible work of our blood cells. Our body contains about twenty trillion red blood cells, and for every 1,000 red blood cells, there is one white blood cell. A drop of blood contains five million red cells and 5,000-10,000 white cells. Red blood cells operate as a vehicle for transporting nutrients and oxygen through the whole body, for feeding and nurturing all tissues and organs of the mind-body.

Red blood cells transport oxygen and nutrient, to all area of mind-body and eliminate carbon dioxide.

- Head
- Lungs
- Heart
- Liver
- Gut
- Rest of the body

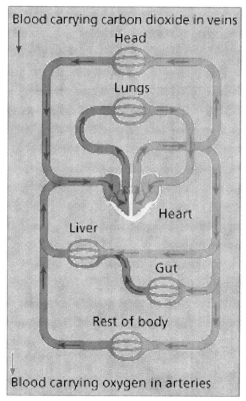

"Taken from CancerHelp UK"

The Bible says life is in the blood (Leviticus 17 : 11). If all the blood is taken from our body, there would have been no more life left in it. The blood never stops flowing through the more than 100,000 km (more than 60,000 miles) of blood vessels (arteries, veins and capillaries), cleansing and feeding each cell, tissue and organ in the body moment by moment. Women average about 4.8 million of these cells per cubic millimeter, men average about 5.4. These values vary. They depend on such factors as health, attitude and environment. The adult human body is producing about 3,000 red blood cells per second. The cells survive about 120 days in the blood before they are destroyed. The bone marrow is constantly reproducing new blood cells to supply the body's need.

Life Begins at 65

Red Blood Cells

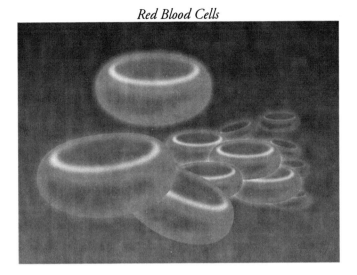

Each hemoglobin molecule of the cell contains over 600 amino acids (amino acids are manufactured from proteins), which have to be laid out according to a precise blueprint and specification designed by the master architect. If even one of the amino acids is placed out of sequence, a fatal disease could result. This is how sickle cell anemia originates. In sickle cell, there is only one amino acid out of its proper sequence, this small deviation could cause illness and may lead to death. What is so fascinating is the team work of the oxygen and the nutrients. They work together in precise sequence. After the delivery of oxygen and nutrients to all the tissues and organs of the body, the waste product of carbon dioxide is collected and transported back to the lungs, to be eliminated. If the carbon dioxide is not eliminated from the body, it will build up to a poisonous level in the cells. Tissues and organs need oxygen and nutrients to stay alive. This is why circulation of the red blood cells is so critical to health.

Low blood platelets (also called thrombocytes) are elements with a fragile membrane. They are one of the three blood groups that provide protection and maintenance for our mind-body. They average about 250,000 - 400,500 per cubic millimeter of blood. They are manufactured in the bone marrow. The rate of their formation seems to depend on the amount of oxygen flowing in the blood and nucleic acid derivative from injured tissue. About one-third of the platelets are located in the spleen. The remaining two-thirds circulate in the blood stream. Their adhesion capabilities allow them to form clots in the blood vessels to prevent excess bleeding if there is an injury to the body. A very low count of platelets could occur as a result of infection, during cancer treatment, or other illnesses.

The white blood cells are soldiers of a finely-tuned immune system that recognizes and destroys foreign substances and organisms that enter the body, protecting us from infections. The immune system can distinguish between the body's own tissues and outside substances known as antigens. The ability of the immune system to identify an antigen permits it to remember antigens that the body has been exposed to in the past so that the soldiers of the immune system can unleash a better and faster immune response the next time any of these "enemy" antigens appear.

Let me take you on a short tour of this incredible system. In this illustration, visualize your mind-body as an island with a white sandy beach surrounded by water. In the water are "terrorist" organisms trying to invade your island. Guarding the island is your defense system. In the water is the first line of defense, the 'infantry and navies'. Granulocytes, monocytes and natural killer cells are on duty. The phagocytes are the neutrophils, basophils and eosinophil; monocyte is the macrophages. Accompanied by the natural killer cells, they hunt down and destroy the 'enemies': organisms, infections, bacteria, parasites, and the like. However, if any of these enemies escape the first line of defense and get on the island, special forces take over. They are the lymphocytes known as T helper cells that send the signal to T killer cells and B plasma cells, to attack the enemies and destroy them. T suppressor cells send signals to stop the attack. When the enemies (antigens) are defeated, B memory cells record their information. If these enemies try to attack again, the defense response will be faster and more efficient. If the T killer cells do not respond to the instruction of the T helper cells to attack the enemies, our island (body) would be over-powered and be taken over by the enemies, who could destroy the island. There is also the danger of communication breakdown between the T suppressor cells and the T killer cells. If the T killer cells do not respond to the instructions of the T suppressor cells, when the enemies are defeated, the T killers must stop their attack. If they continue to attack, they will start destroying good cells. In the army, when soldiers are accidentally killed by their own team members, it is called friendly fire. In the immune system this is referred to as autoimmune disease.

Our defense system is given to us by our Creator to protect and heal us when we get sick. We need to supply it with the essential nutrients it needs.

My advice to all cancer survivors is that life is what one makes it. Courage, hope, faith, sympathy, forgiveness and love promote and prolong life and strength to the soul. "A merry (rejoicing) heart doeth good like a medicine" Proverbs 17:22 (KJ).

My studies in nutrition provide me with the understanding that if cancer is present, there are many points during the development stages in which nutrition and lifestyle changes can be an important factor. In fact, there are some nutrients that will inhibit cancer at the initiation and promotion stage, deactivating the cancer and strengthening the immune system.

All diseases are curable, but not all people. It is all up to the individual. We can read hundreds of testimonials from people who did the impossible without their doctors, but the reality is that they changed their life and lifestyle. Real healing is not just a quick fix. If we want to be healthy and joyful, we have to address the reason why we are sick. There is no such thing as "once healed always healed." Healing is a constant process and must integrate mind and body.

We have a flood of messenger molecules coursing through the bloodstream, transforming our most intimate thoughts, emotional beliefs, prejudices, wishes, dreams, choices, and fears into physical reality. Reality is a conscious process of our emotional reactions to life and health. The cause of many illnesses can be traced back to some physical, mental, spiritual, or emotional imbalance in our life. If we take time to research the past performance of our mind-body, we could likely diagnose where many of our illnesses began. We need to become more aware of subtle warning messages that often tell us that something is wrong. Many of us often ignore warning signs until they become chronic diseases. We need to develop a conscious habit of listening to our mind-body. We cannot experience the faintest emotion without our heart cells sharing it with our lungs, kidneys, stomach, and intestines. Thoughts translate themselves into physiological effects that are critical to health and wellness. The physical is the foundation for the human existence. It is the house we live in. It provides the operation of the mental powers, and the mental powers provide for the highest operation in us, the spiritual dimension.

During my eleven-day stay in hospital, my wife was there every day to see me. Many of the days the weather was unpleasant, and she had to drive from Scarborough to Whitby to work after her visits. My pastors, church family, relatives and friends visited and called me on the phone. This brought joy to my heart. Lying on my back in the hospital bed, I was inspired by the reality that love is the greatest incentive to a new start in our journey of life. It is the purest of all incentives. Love never gives up on its object of affection. My wife's love, demonstrated by action, inspires and stimulates me. More than that, the life-giving blood of Christ flows through my whole body to provide healing. This is what this world needs for true healing. Love motivates hope and trust in our Creator. It provides the incentive for a more caring society, where governments and companies will spend more money on health care to save lives, and less money on war, that destroys lives. Many of our illnesses are created from fear, hate, prejudice, greed, selfishness, and other similar negative emotions. Many people have lost faith in government and our health care system. We need a health care system that is proactive rather than reactive. As a society, we need to recreate that atmosphere of love where faith and hope will alleviate fear.

All patients, whether they are fighting a disease or managing a chronic condition, live in hope of new medicines and improved therapies. Are we meeting these hopes with new medications and treatment options? Disease is our common enemy! Treatment given by our physicians and health care professionals should always reflect the patient's need. As we search for new cures to alleviate pain and suffering, let's focus on what is best for suffering humanity and not what is profitable for drug companies. A recent poll taken by USA Today and public opinion researchers at the Kaiser Family Foundation and Harvard School of Public Health, finds that Americans greatly value prescription drugs' potential benefits for their families, but most believed they cost too much money. Many of these families are struggling to pay for needed medication. Are we at war with disease, or are we taking disadvantage of the sick, helpless and vulnerable people of our society? These are fundamental questions we need to answer, as we make health care plans for our society, and our future generation.

Although government policies dictate our formal health care system, each of us must take personal responsibility to educate ourselves and our society about the significance of healthy living. When we take action to evaluate our lifestyle, we will realize that sickness is not a period that ends this great sentence of life, it a comma that punctuates it to a conscious awareness of the need to make healthy lifestyle changes as we continue life's journey.

There is also the need for the understanding that sometimes death is a welcome friend! I know; it was a relief to my father and brother-in-law. My mother told me she regularly prayed that my father's enduring suffering during his illness would come to an end, to relieve him of his agonizing pain. My brother-in-law went through a similar experience. Within three months of being diagnosesd with prostate cancer, his ribs started collapsing. It's difficult to lose loved ones who are so dear to you. I truly miss my father. He was very special. I loved him very much. I also loved my brother-in-law. This is why folks should understand that when we have a strong faith in our Creator, death will not be a blind alley that leads to an unknown destination. It will be an open highway that leads to a city, where there will be no more sickness, no pain, no fear of death and no fear of the unknown. All these conditions will be in the past. There will be everlasting joy, contentment, peace and serenity. Having this wonderful hope, I do not worry about death. I use my time and energy planning how to love and help others in their time of need.

I recall that many years ago I went into hiding after my surgery for prostate cancer. I had lost my job as Chief Engineer with the Ministry of Education so I took a job as a Building Superintendent, because I thought I was too old to compete in the job market. I sold my home and took this job, with the intention of getting a free apartment for my wife and myself. I was surrendering my will to compete. I was hiding from reality. Three months into the job, while babysitting tenants, I realized, this was not for me. So I left that job, and took a course as a healthcare worker. I completed the course within three months and got three part-time jobs with three hospitals. That motivated me to apply for an engineering position. I got the job, which resulted in a change in my thought process. This is why I strongly recommend to people who find themselves in a depressive mood, to become more proactive. Worrying about age, sickness or death depletes your energy, weakens your major response systems and subjects your mind-body to degenerative diseases, which are plaguing our society. My whole perspective of this journey of life has been changed. We have to make choices, and these choices will affect how we meander the difficult terrains as we continue our journey of life.

I continue to emphasize these thoughts and experiences because age and sickness can be tools to enhance our success of health and wealth. By developing a renewed perspective, sickness can, in fact, rekindle a new start in life's fascinating journey. I see from the male perspective that men are becoming an endangered species. It seems to me that we as men generally reach a destination where we disregard our right to think and make relevant choices about where our life's journey will end. We have become so complacent, so dependent on technology and the news media that we allow them to make decisions about our health choices. We have ignored our mind-body cries for help. Are we conscious of the environment around us, and how deviant our society is becoming? We're being exploited by the very systems that should be taking care of us. The warning signals are telling us to slow down; relax; take some time to visualize and assess our surroundings. We were created to serve and be served; to love and be loved. Sin has caused our world to deteriorate. God, in his infinite mercy and wisdom, has provided us with the ability to withstand and evaluate many of the dangerous terrains we encounter in life's journey. We need to be proactive about the warning signals. The relationship between our mind-body, our environment, and our emotionional behaviors dictate our survival.

Walter Cannon, a professor of physiology at Harvard University, looked at the need for mental and physical balance throughout organism, and coined the term 'Homeostasis', from the Greek word homoios, meaning similar, and stasis, meaning position. In his work with animals, Cannon observed the change and state of emotion in animals. These include distress, rage, anxiety, fear, and depression, accompanied by total cessation of the stomach. What affects the stomach affects the whole body. Cannon's study into the relationship between the effect of emotions and perceptions on the autonomic nervous system took into account both sympathetic and parasympathetic responses. He concluded that the effects initiate fight or flight responses. These are everyday experiences and challenges. We would do well to learn how to identify these effects so we can make positive decisions in a timely way.

Emulating Cannon's work, Hans Selye experimented with animals. He subjected them to conditions offering different physical and mental stressors and noted that under these adverse conditions, the body constantly adapted to heal and recover. Like animals, humans can become adapted to adverse environmental conditions. However, these situations and conditions placed great demand on our cells, organs and systems. As we grow older, we have to learn how to cope with these changes. Many of us have migrated from different countries to North America. Our lifestyles and diets are different in many ways. Some researchers have suggested that the risk for prostate cancer increases for some nationalities when they migrate to North America. Men need to know this type of information so they can make better decisions and take preventative measures to alleviate these risk factors. Many of us search for answers through human experiences that elevate and unite our thoughts and feelings. As we begin to better understand life's complexities and the relevance of our experiences, only then are we able to make decisions that will alleviate negative stressors that suppress our health. We must replace such stressors with more positive actions that serve to enhance our health.

Humans have a tendency to respond with anger and aggression to perception of danger. Many of these dangers do not allow for a fight or flight response. For example, a worker might perceive that he or she is being unfairly persecuted by the supervisor. The worker might be afraid that if she's assertive in responding to her boss, her employment will be terminated., So what does she do? She suppresses her feelings. This can cause chronic stress that leads to severe depression and disease. Be proactive rather than reactive!

On April 18, 2008, I celebrate my 68th birthday. I thank God for the good health I'm enjoying. From 2005 to 2007 I worked in construction in the Alberta oil fields. From spring through fall I worked as a pipefitter while studying for my doctor of science in nutrition. Many of the workers were surprised at my physical performance. I have also completed my PhD in nutrition. In my journey of life, I am living one day at a time and enjoying God's abundant blessings. Every day is a new beginning for me, with new experiences. With a wonderful wife to love, and who loves me, life does begin at 65. Prostate, or any cancer, does not have to control your life. You are in control. So, men, let's talk about the prostate and see if we can learn something about this little gland that can become a big problem. Or it can be no problem.

Chapter 2:
An Overview of Prostate

The prostate, a sex gland found only in men, is located inside the lower abdomen at the base of the penis, just below the bladder and in front of the rectum. The word "prostate" comes from the Greek word *prohistani* meaning standing in front of. The prostate gland is a small organ about the size of a chestnut. The urethra, the channel that carries urine from the bladder and through the penis, runs through prostate. The prostate gland is one of the body parts that most men rarely think about; that is, until they begin to have problems. The primary function of the prostate gland is to secrete fluid and vital nutrients and semen, the milky ejaculate that nourishes sperm, which are produced by the testicles. The sperm travels up from the testicles through long tubes called the vas deferens.

The prostate located below the bladder and surrounds the Urethra.

- Ureters
- Bladder
- Prostate
- Urethra

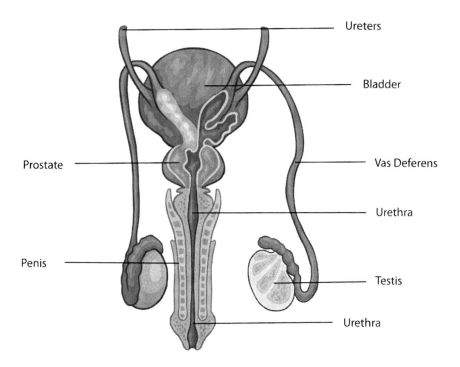

During orgasm, the prostate fluid mixes with fluid from the seminal vesicles, located on each side of the prostate. One specific function of the prostatic fluid is to regulate the acidity of semen as it travels through the acid environment of the female reproductive tract. Special muscles squeeze the fluid into the urethra, where it carries sperm through the penis during orgasm. To make sure semen doesn't move in the wrong direction and back up into the bladder, a ring of muscle at the neck of the bladder (the internal sphincter) remains tightened during ejaculation.

The prostate wraps completely around the urethra, the tube that empties urine from the bladder through the penis; it is at a position that leads to difficulties later in life. In newborns the prostate is about the size of a pea. It continues to grow until about age twenty, when it reaches the normal adult size of a walnut. It is suggested by researchers that it remains that size until, on average, age forty-five, at which time it begins to grow again, as testosterone levels began to decline.

Another view of the prostate

- Bladder
- Prostate Gland
- Penis
- Urethra
- Testis

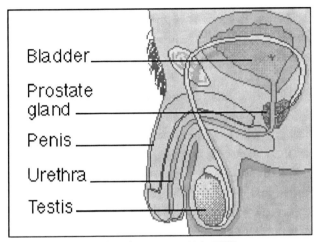

"Taken from CancerHelp UK"

The prostate veins drain toward the heart via connections along the spine. Lymph, a watery fluid found in all tissues, flows away from the prostate via smart channels (lymphatic) to lymph nodes, which filter out bacteria, viruses, and other impurities as well as cancer cells before the lymph flows further up stream toward veins that eventually empty into the heart. This would suggest that, if there are physical or other problems with the operation with the lymphatic system, infection or disease could be the result. The prostate is part of the urinary and reproductive system; some health professionals believe it is not a vital organ, but from my experience, it is. All organs are important to the efficient operation of mind and body; because a person can live without a specific organ doesn't mean that it should be taken out. Because some of our doctors do not understand the real purpose of the organ does not alleviate its importance. Our Creator designed every part in our system for a special reason. My experience as an engineer tells me that when a piece of equipment is being repaired the technician doesn't discard a part because he doesn't know how it works and the equipment can operate without it. The technician would be compromising the safe and efficient operation of the equipment. Humans are more important than machines. My personal experience teaches me that when a person loses a vital organ, it cannot be replaced by an artificial man-made organ and operate without health problems.

The prostate may be small, but it is a complicated organ. It contains two main kinds of tissue: the smooth muscle and hundreds of tiny, spongy glands. Because it has these two different kinds of tissue, the prostate is sometimes described as a musculoglandular structure.

The outer coat, by which most of the prostate is surrounded, has a thick fibrous membrane sometimes called the capsule. The prostate is divided into three zones. Seventy percent of the zones are the prostate's glandular tissue. The rest of the glandular tissues are found in the smaller central and transition zones completely surrounding the urethra and are usually the smallest of the three zones. The other major region of the prostate is the anterior tissue, which is mostly made up of smooth muscle and is not usually involved in prostatic disease.

The prostate lies in close proximity to other tissues and organs, and its function is intimately connected with theirs. As previously mentioned, the urethra passes through the middle of the prostate, as do the ejaculatory ducts from the seminal vesicles. The prostate is located under the bladder, directly in front of the rectum. All these structures are kept alive and nourished by the delicate and complex network of nerves and blood vessels. Nerves that run alongside the prostate, contained within the neurovascular bundles, are responsible for making the penis become hard during an erection. The presence of all these tissues complicates treatment choices enormously, because therapies that are focused on that area may have indirect unwanted effects on other areas. Removing the erectile nerves, for example, means naturally occurring erection are no longer possible.

Hormone is the chemical messenger that makes the prostate grows. In childhood the prostate is about the size of a pea; during puberty the body begins producing large amounts of male hormones or androgens, which cause the prostate to grow more rapidly, into its full size and shape. The most important form of androgen is testosterone. Most testosterone, about 95 percent, is produced by the testicles. It is suggested by doctors that triggering of prostate growth is just one function of androgens. These powerful chemicals also control all aspects of the body change known as virilization (growth of the scrotum, testicles, penis, development of body hair, deepening of the voice, and increase in muscle bulk, especially in the chest and shoulders). Androgens also cause the prostate to begin manufacturing prostatic fluid.

Once the prostate reaches normal adult size, it generally stops growing until men reach middle age. At that point it often starts to enlarge even more, probably because of the complex hormonal changes associated with aging. Over time, an enlarged prostate may start to squeeze the urethra, affecting a man's ability to urinate. This glandular increase in the size of the prostate leads to a condition that could cause problem for some men later in life.

The action of the testosterone on the prostate is part of complex change and biochemical events. First a tiny gland in the brain, the hypothalamus, pumps out luteinizing hormone- releasing hormone (LHRH). The LHRH travels to the nearby pituitary to secrete hormones known as gonadotropins (the word basically means "chemical that turns on the gonads"). One of the gonadotropins is luteinizing hormone (LH). LH circulates to the testicles, which respond by releasing testosterone into the blood stream. Once in circulation some of the testosterone travels to the prostate, where it is absorbed by individual prostate cells. Inside the cell an enzyme called alpha-reductase converts the testosterone into dihydrotestosterone, or DHT. The DHT then migrates to the cell's nucleus, where it begins doing its work.

Endocrine glands that control hormones

- Pinal
- Pituitary
- Thyroid

- Parathyroids…

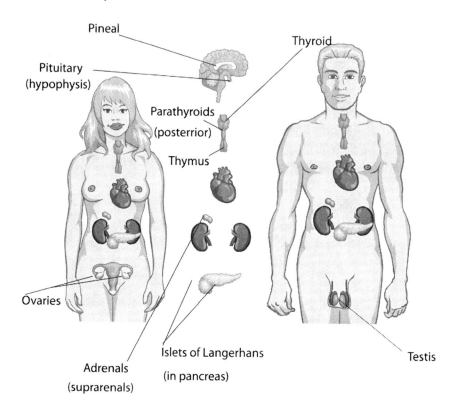

In addition to the androgens produced by the testicles, some androgens are produced by the adrenal glands in both men and women. In response to hormonal signals from the hypothalamus, the pituitary gland secretes a substance called adrenocorticotropic hormone (ACTH). This hormone travels to the adrenal glands and stimulates them to produce adrenal androgens, which are not as powerful as the androgen produced by the testicles. For example, they don't usually cause virilization unless abnormally large amounts are produced. Besides driving prostate growth, androgen is assumed to fuel the growth of prostate cancer cells, similar to the way gasoline fuels fire.

Because of the way the prostate surrounds the urethra, prostate disease can have a major impact on urination. To understand the problem, here's a quick guided tour of the male urinary system.

The urinary tract begins with the kidneys, two bean-shaped organs roughly the size of your fists that lie on either side of the spine at the bottom of the rib cage. The kidneys filter out toxic wastes, excess water, and salts from the blood. At the same time they salvage useful materials and recycle them into the blood stream. In the average man, the kidneys produce about two quarts of urine per day. The urine drains into the muscular tubes called the urethras, which squeeze the urine out of the kidneys, pushing it down into the bladder and forming a one-way-valve mechanism that prevent urine from flowing back into the kidneys.

The kidneys filter out toxic wastes, excess water, and salts from the blood stream.

- The Kidneys
- The Urinary System

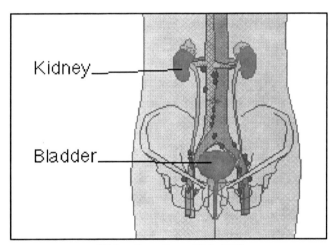

"Taken from CancerHelp UK"

The bladder is basically a muscular reservoir for urine. As it fills, the bladder expands; and as it empties it contracts. When the system is healthy and functioning, a man can choose when he want to eliminate urine. Problems with the muscle in the bladder or other urinary structures, however, can reduce the ability to regulate urination, and as a result urine can dribble or leak out.

Urine flows from the bladder unto the urethra, a tube that is about eight inches long and tunnels through the prostate at an angle and then travels down through the penis. If the prostate becomes enlarged, the urethra may be constricted or narrowed, preventing urine from flowing properly. Besides being part of the urinary tract, the prostate forms part of the male reproductive system, which also includes the testicles, the epididymis, the vas deferens, the seminal vesicles, the ejaculatory ducts, and the penis.

Problems in the prostate or any of these other urinary parts can impair fertility. They can also interfere with the ability to have an erection or to experience orgasms and ejaculation.

The testicles, which get their blood supply from a vessel known as the testicular artery in the spermatic cord, are responsible for the production of sperm. Immature sperm are manufactured in hundreds of tiny compartments or tubules within the testicles. Then they migrate by the millions to the epididymis, where they mature. The testicles are also the main source of testosterone, which it is suggested by doctors stimulates tumor growth. In the case of prostate disease, strategies to eliminate testosterone include the use of drugs that block its production or the surgical removal of the testicles.

The penis is a complex structure made up of nerves, smooth muscle, and blood vessels. It becomes erect by a well-engineered system. Under normal conditions, sexual stimulation causes the nerves in the penis to instruct the arteries to expand and to retain extra blood. The nerves then signal the veins to constrict so that the blood comes in but cannot flow out as quickly. As the blood fills up the three hollow, spongy tissue structures in the penis, erection occurs. Many of the nerves that control erection run along either side of the prostate. If cancer cells penetrate the prostate and enter the nerves on one or both sides, the nerves must be removed during surgery.

Chapter 3:
Prostate Disorder Diagnosis and Treatment

As stated in chapter two, the prostate is a small gland, a part of the lower urinary system in men and primarily reproductive in function. Along with the testicles and seminal vesicles, the prostate sits below the urinary bladder and surrounds the upper part of the urethra, the tube that carries urine from the bladder.

There are three major diseases that can affect the prostate:

- Prostatitis, an inflammatory disease
- Benign prostate hyperplasia (BPH), most commonly a disease of aging
- Prostate cancer, the second most common cancer in men today

PROSTATITIS

It is suggested by some health professionals that prostatitis is one of the most neglected diseases in North America. It strikes more men than either prostate cancer or prostate enlargement does. It can be one of the most miserable diseases inflicted on men. It does not discriminate, it could strikes at a young age, and it lasts longer than many diseases.

Urologists estimate that one in every four men who see a doctor about a problem involving the penis, urethra, testicles, prostate, bladder, or kidneys is suffering from one of these types of the disease. Prostatitis is not a threat to life, and for practical purposes, research for treatment for prostatitis is limited or does not exist. Drug companies do not invest in research projects that do not provide lucrative profit.

The symptoms of prostatitis are a frequent urge to urinate, difficult start, dribbling, night trips to the bathroom, fever, decreased libido or impotence, painful ejaculation, low-back pain, and perineal pain. The symptom that sets prostatitis apart from prostate growth is pain. This varies from mild to severe and can render a man helpless. Some people refer to a man in severe prostatitis pain as a "prostate cripple." A man with the symptoms just listed usually has acute prostatitis, inflammation of the prostate caused by bacteria, which often afflicts young men. Physical examination often fails to clarify the cause of the pain. Cultures and microscopic examination of urine and prostatic secretions before and after prostatic massage may help differentiate prostatitis caused by infection from prostatitis with other causes. Acute bacterial prostatitis is said to hit hard and fast. Acute bacterial prostatitis is like any other major bacterial infection in the body, but it happens to be localized in the prostate. Because the infection is centered in the prostate, men may have pain anywhere below the belt, all the way through to the back and down to the genitals, frequency of urination, incomplete voiding of the bladder, or even a complete inability to urinate. My experience after prostate cancer surgery qualifies me to say I understand the painful situation a man experience when he has problem voiding his urine.

The process by which men get bacterial prostatitis is the same as with any other infection. Bacteria enters the body and, if not destroyed by the immune system, will instead "settle down" in the prostate. The infection may have arrived through the urethra via the urinary tract, or perhaps it might have spread from an infection elsewhere in the body via the bloodstream.

In order to make a diagnosis of acute bacterial prostatitis, the doctors will note the general symptoms and insert a finger into the man's rectum to probe the prostate. The doctor can massage the prostate with the finger to allow the prostatic fluid to be pushed into the urethra and out of the tip of the penis. Microscopic examination of the prostatic fluid can be undertaken to test for the offending bacteria. The problem with these tests is that doctors are concentrating on a specific organ or symptom and not the cause of the infection. The prostate is located in the line of one of the five elimination organs that are critical to optimum health and wellness. Infection could be caused by lack of proper elimination of the urinary system.

The conventional treatment for acute bacterial prostatitis is usually antibiotics and bed rest, plus intravenous fluids and other medicines the doctor might think necessary. Most times the medications work by suppressing symptoms to relieve the pain; sometimes they don't. If unchecked, acute bacterial prostatitis could lead to serious problems such as abscesses in the prostate or chronic bacterial prostatitis, etc. The proper way to cure an illness is to treat the whole body, not just the symptom.

Like the acute version, chronic bacterial prostatitis is inflammation of the prostate caused by bacteria, but the chronic form generally produces few symptoms, although the symptoms last much longer. Probably, the bacteria settles into the prostate for longer because the method of treatments were ineffective. The immune system may have prevented the germs from spreading too far, or doing too much damage, but it failed to get rid of them entirely. It is suggested that diagnosing chronic bacterial prostatitis can be difficult because the symptoms are less severe. The afflicted man may suffer from urgency, frequent urination, excessive nighttime urination, pain upon urination, or difficulty urinating. The symptoms may lessen or disappear for a while, only to return again. The fact that a man has the same infection over and over again is an important clue for the doctors to assess the problem.

As usual conventional treatment involves the use of antibiotics such as Cipro (Ciprofloxacin), Maxaquin (Hydrochloride), and Tetracycline.

If the response to the therapy relieves the symptoms, antibiotics are continued for at least three to four weeks, although some men are given treatment for several months. Doctors suggest that while the drugs seem to be good at taking care of acute bacterial infections, they are not effective against chronic prostatitis because they don't penetrate well into the prostate. Doctors fail to understand that antibiotic is not the only treatment for infections. There are alternative treatments that have been researched, proven, and recorded in nutritional and other natural treatment journals. Treatment therapies should be tailored to provide healing for the sick patient, not for the relieving of symptoms.

The third form of prostatitis is said to be nonbacterial: Bacteria do not seem to be too involved, although the symptoms are similar to those of bacterial prostatitis. Laboratory examination of fluids massaged out of the prostate may show an increased number of white blood cells, suggestive of a problem of some sort, but bacteria can't always be found in the samples. Doctors believe bacteria are not the cause, or that some bacteria that elude identification are responsible.

Although doctors do not know what does cause nonbacterial prostatitis, they do know that it is often found in young, sexually active men. They suspect that the cause of the problem occurs during sexual transmission.

Although evidence to support the following recommendations are limited, physicians may consider a diagnostic test, such as a four-glass test or the PPMT. In most cases, empiric antibiotic therapy is considered to be reasonable, whether or not the diagnostic test proves a bacterial cause. Common choices include TMP-SMX, doxycycline, or one of the fluoroquinolones. Treatment is often recommended for four weeks, although some clinicians use shorter courses. It is suggested that physicians should encourage hydration, which treats pain appropriately, and consider the use of NSAIDs, an alpha-blocking agent, or both. If symptoms persist, a more thorough evaluation for CNP/CPPS should be pursued. Some men may need several trials of different therapies to find one that alleviates their symptoms.

Doctors have the same problem treating nonbacterial prostatitis, because they don't know what causes it. However, antibiotics are tried for treatment, with trial of other medicines. The term prostatitis describes a wide spectrum of conditions with variable etiologies, prognoses, and treatments. Unfortunately, these conditions have not been well studied, and most recommendations for treatment, including those given here, are based primarily on case series and anecdotal experience. For these reasons, many men and their physicians find prostatitis to be a challenging condition to be treated. The problem with this method of treatment is that long-term antibiotics therapy could damage the good flora in the digestive system and could lead to other complications. Sometimes, hot water or hot whirlpool baths lasting for about twenty minutes are also used as temporary relief.

BENIGN PROSTATIC HYPERPLASIA (BPH)

The prostate usually begins to enlarge in almost all men in their forties. Researchers suggest that once growth starts, it does not stop as long as life goes on. Effects of this growth vary from almost unbearable misery to minor annoyance, The general rule is that one in four men over age sixty will become so burdened by BPH that he will need physical relief. The prostate begins to enlarge through a process of cell multiplication called benign prostatic hyperplasia (BPH). The symptoms of BPH can mirror late-stage prostate cancer because the enlarging inner portion of the prostate puts pressure on the urethra, which can potentially cause urinary problems.

Why doctors label this condition "benign" is difficult to understand. If the BPH is not properly cared for, it can lead to extremely serious consequences, including kidney damage and failure. It is important to know that the prostate grows in two different ways. In one kind of growth, cells multiply around the urinary passageway within the prostate and squeeze the urethra. The second type of growth is much worse; this is a middle growth in which cells grow into the urine tube and even up and into the bladder. It is suggested by doctors that this type of growth can be cleared up only through surgery. The most effective surgical procedures, transurethral resection of the prostate (TURP) and open prostatectomy, are also the most invasive. They carry the highest risks for significant complications, including impotence and incontinence. Because of the invasiveness of surgery, it is imperative that when a man is considering treatment he should be sure his surgeon performs at least fifty of these procedures each year. It is suggested that the complication rates of the surgeon should be no higher than 1 percent for incontinence and 4 percent for impotence.

Cell growth into the urine tube and the bladder suggest that prostate enlargement is not simply a case of too many prostate cells. This growth involves hormones; it involves different kinds of prostate cells; and it affects each man differently. As a result of these differences, the medical professionals believe that nothing answers growth problems for every man. "Nothing" refers to the well-known "Roto Rooter" operation, to drugs, to heat treatments, and to drug-free substances. The medical professionals believe that there is no cure for prostate growth; they believe that once it starts it never stops.

People sometimes ask if an enlargement of the prostate increases the risk of prostate cancer. The medical community suggests that there is no connection. A man can have prostate growth with no cancer. He can have prostate growth with cancer, and he can have prostate cancer without enlargement. Conventional medicine treatment options have increased: They are (1) surgery; (2) procedures similar to surgery but considered "noninvasive" or minimally invasive; (3) prescription medicines; and (4) two other available treatments, which are used as "last resort." One is dilation of the urine passageway. The second is cryoablation, or cryotherapy, which freezes the prostate. Because this procedure was associated with significant side effects, it was abandoned until the early 1990s. With the introduction of transrectal ultrasound (TRUS), monitoring of probe placement and freezing was achieved.

Surgery: Many years ago, surgery included the cleaning out of the prostate through the bladder by retropubic operation, which was not appropriate for all men. Timing is vital when considering surgery for BPH; therefore it's imperative that men discuss their symptoms and the effect those symptoms have on their lives and the lives of their families. Retropubic procedure means the removal of either part or all of the prostate gland. Most doctors recommended early operations, because the risk of kidney damage was much increased if the symptoms were gradually getting worse. However, these procedures have been almost entirely replaced by more advanced techniques introduced by the medical community.

TUIP (Trans-Urethral Incision of the Prostate): The physician inserts a cutting instrument through the prostate to reach the neck of the bladder. He makes two large lengthwise cuts to tissue from the neck of the bladder and through the length of the prostate. This procedure is similar to TURP except that rather than removing the tissue, one or two small incisions are made in the prostate, causing the bladder neck and the prostate to open and relieve pressure on the urethra. It is suggested that men who are interested in having children should consider it because it does not affect ejaculation or fertility provided the prostate is one ounce or smaller.

TURP (Trans-Urethral Resection of the Prostate): It is suggested that in the 1980s TURP accounted for about 95 percent of all prostate surgery, but it has declined as alternatives procedures have become more widely available. Some urologists still think of it as "the Gold Standard" in treating prostate enlargement. While in general this procedure is recognized by doctors to be safe, patients require spinal, epidural, or general anesthesia and also need days of hospitalization and weeks of recovery. The potential for morbidity and mortality limits the use of TURP in patients with high surgical risk. Potential complication include bleeding, infection, and prolonged catheterization as well as the frequent need for a repeat operation. If the fluids used during TURP build up, water intoxication can develop, which can be serious. Symptoms including abdominal cramps, nausea, vomiting, lethargy, and dizziness and are referred to as TURP syndrome. In this procedure, after the patient is anaesthetized, the urologist inserts a resectoscope into the penis and passes it along the urethra until it reaches the bladder neck. The urologist then uses an electric cutting loop on the end of the resectoscope to cut away the enlarged tissue of the inner portion of the prostate.

Transurethral Needle Ablation of the Prostate (TUNA): TUNA is referred as a simple, safe, and relatively inexpensive procedure. The doctors uses needles to deliver high-frequency radio waves (microwaves) that heat and create lesions within the prostate to destroy excess prostate tissue. The procedure only requires topical urethral anesthesia. It is believed to be less effective than TURP. The technique is similar to indigo laser and other noninvasive techniques and works best on the moderately enlarged prostate, though it is not very effective on very large ones.

A study found that symptoms improved after six months. Complications include urinary retention, blood in the urine, retrograde ejaculation, and painful urination. However, it appears to pose very low to no risk of incontinence and impotence.

Laser Surgery: Various transurethral laser techniques have been developed and are being used in removing excess prostate tissue or vaporizing it. This approach uses laser energy direct with a fiber via a cyst scope into the prostate and uses heat to shrink the gland. This procedure is faster than TURP and causes no bleeding. There are two disadvantages of laser techniques: There is prolonged cauterization during the postoperative phase and no tissue is obtained during the procedure. In roller-ball laser surgery, direct contact with prostate tissue vaporizes it. In this procedure, the "laser-induced" and "laser-assisted" surgery, high-energy instruments heat prostate tissue to as high as 140 to 212 degrees. It is suggested by researchers that this heat kills the tissue and the body throws it off.

Indigo-Laser: The physician inserts a needle-shaped probe into the prostate and then fires energy in the shape of a ball from the probe's tip. The blast of the heat destroys prostate tissue. This is relatively recent therapy. The manufacturer sells its results favourable to "Gold-Standard" TURP. However, it is suggested that this procedure is too new for one to be sure of its long-term value.

Transurethral Microwave Thermotherapy (TUMT): This procedure, which was approved by the FDA in May 1996, is referred to as the "Granddaddy" of heat therapy for prostate enlargement. It includes a device that uses microwaves to heat and destroy excess prostate tissue. In this procedure, a prostatron-regulated microwave antenna is inserted through the urethra with ultrasound used to position it accurately. The antenna is enclosed in a cooling tube to protect the lining of the urethra. Computer-generated microwaves pulse through the antenna to heat selected portions of the prostate to about 111 degrees Fahrenheit. A cooling system protects the urinary tract during the procedure.

Transurethral Electrovaporization (TUEVP): This procedure uses high voltage to combine vaporization of prostate tissue and coagulation, which seals the blood and lymph vessels around the area. The excess tissue, deprived of blood, dies and is sloughed off over time. A study suggested that patients who had TUEVP were able to have their catheter removed fourteen to sixteen hours after the procedure compared to normal removal time of three to five days after TURP. The average hospital stay was only nineteen to thirty-six hours.

Hot-Water Therapy: The device known as thermoflex, which circulates heated water through a catheter to destroy prostatic tissue, has been approved for treating BPH. There is also another technique that uses a balloon filled with water to destroy tissue around the urethra. The procedure does not require anesthesia and can be completed during an outpatient visit.

Open Prostatectomy: In open prostatectomy the enlarged prostate is removed through an open incision in the abdomen using standard surgical techniques. This is said to be a major surgery and requires a hospital stay of several days. This procedure is only used for severe cases, in about 2 percent to 3 percent of patients, when the prostate is severely enlarged, and the bladder could be damaged; other potential serious problems exist. It is suggested that up to 14 percent of patients require a second operation because of scarring. In making a decision about open prostatectomy and discussing the consequences, it is imperative that BPH men be assertive. Physicians have the responsibility to advise patients of the side effects of a diminished sexual capacity, which can often occur after this procedure. Prostatectomy should be considered as a last resort.

Prostatic Stent: Prostatic stent is a procedure where urolume, a mesh-like flexible tube made of a special alloy, is inserted into the urethra, where it expands and eases urine flow. The tube does not cause reaction in the body. The procedure takes only fifteen minutes and requires only regional anesthetic and mild sedation. Patients require minimal recuperation and no overnight hospital stay.

Prostatron Treatment: This system uses cooled thermo therapy, otherwise known an transurethral microwave thermotherapy (TUMT) to deliver precisely targeted microwave energy to heat and destroy hyperplastic prostate tissue. At the same time, a unique cooling mechanism protects the surrounding healthy tissue, creating coagulative necrosis. Cooling water is circulated through outer channels of the catheter for protection of the urethra edema, for faster patient recovery. Prostatron was approved by the FDA in 1996 as an alternative treatment for enlarged prostate.

Tragis System: Approved by the FDA in September 1997, similar to the prostatron this procedure delivers microwaves to destroy selected portions of the prostate and a cooling system to protect the urethra. A heat-sensing device inserted in the rectum helps monitor the therapy. Both procedures take about one hour and can be performed at an outpatient basis without general anesthesia. It is suggested that neither procedure has been reported as the cause of impotence or incontinence. Microwave therapy does not cure BPH; it reduces urinary frequency, urgency, straining, and intermittent flow. It does not correct the problem of incomplete emptying of the bladder.

ORAL ALTERNATIVES TO SURGERY

Hytrin, Gardura, Flomax: These prescription drugs were originally developed to relax heart muscles. Experiments by doctors found that they also relax prostate muscles, which relieves the pressure on the urine channel through the prostate. Research claims that they help about 70 percent of men who try them. Side effects include lowering blood pressure and dizziness. Flomax, the newest of the three, is suggested by doctors to have fewer side effects.

Proscar: This drug shrinks the tissue around the prostate's urine channel and the prostate itself. It is controversial. Information gathered by the American Prostate Society suggests that it helps about one in three men, and it takes about ten months for any benefits to appear.

Men today have many options in seeking relief from the symptoms of prostate growth. It is up to every man to consider all options based on his personal needs. Men should not rely on their doctor to do this for them. If your doctor specializes in TUMT, you will not get TUNA as an option. If he is partial to TURP and "Roto-Rooter," he may choose surgery. In treating prostate growth you are not likely to receive a prescription for an oral drug, not to mention anything for relief in alternative or natural treatment, from most standard physicians.

Prostate Cancer

Thirdly, there is prostate cancer. Prostate cancer is the most common cancer in men today. Canadian men have a one in nine chance of developing this disease. It is also the second leading cause of cancer death in men. It is estimated that 17,800 men in Canada will be diagnosed this year with prostate cancer, and 4,300 will die of this disease. Approximately 189,000 American men were expected to be diagnosed with prostate cancer in 2002 compared to 165,000 in 1993. Also in 2002, 30,000 American men were predicted to die of prostate cancer. Approximately 3 percent of all deaths of American men are currently believed to be caused by prostate cancer. This is a large number of people, but it means that only 3 men in 100 will actually die of the disease, which if detected and treated early can provide men an excellent chance of recovery. Fortunately, prostate cancer is a slow-growing disease, in most cases, giving some men time to make the correct treatment choice for themselves. The idea that it is a slow-growing cancer has proven to cause the death of some men, because they misjudge the aggressiveness of the cancer growth. Therefore, because of the life-or-death situation involve with prostate cancer, every man must be properly informed and educated so that he will be in a position to make a proper decision.

Prostate cancer compressing urethra

- The tumor growth presses on the urethra
- Blocks the flow of urine

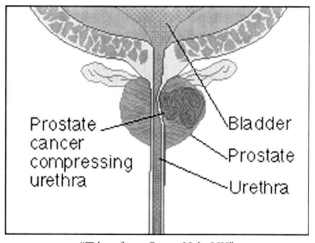

"Taken from CancerHelp UK"

Prostate cancer tends to affect men over the age of fifty. Though prostate cancer is more rare in men under the age of fifty, it can be more aggressive and faster growing in younger men. The presence of prostate cancer cells is surprising common in men of all age groups. Autopsy studies have shown that cancer cells can be detected within the prostate in 26 percent of men aged thirty to forty years and 38 percent of men in their fifties. Prostate cancer cells seem to exist either as latent cancers whose numbers expand very slowly, which seems to be the situation in 85 percent of men, or as actively growing cancers with the ability and propensity to metastasize. Researchers have suggested that the cause for this change in behaviour of a slow-growing latent cancer to an aggressive carcinoma is not clear, but at present it is a subject of investigation. They theorize that a family history of prostate cancer is a strong risk factor, and that men with one or more first-degree relatives—father and brothers—have a higher risk. Black men are also at an increased risk of prostate cancer. In these two groups it is recommended that screening start at age forty. For others, the Canadian Urological Association recommends a yearly digital rectal exam beginning at age fifty.

However, studies indicate that the global difference in incidences is not totally due to genetics. If individuals with the same genetic background are reared in different environments, the risk of developing prostate cancer is associated with the country in which they reside. Examples of changes in cancer risk associated with reverse migration have been reported. Less aggressive forms of cancer tend to develop in low-risk countries. Incidents of prostate cancer increase from three to sevenfold in first generation Chinese American, Japanese American, and African American men compared to Chinese, Japanese, and African men still living in their homelands.

Per capita fat consumption has been linked to the development of prostate cancer and the death rate from this disease. The United States, Canada, Western European countries, and Jamaica have the highest death rates from prostate cancer and the highest per capita fat consumption. In contrast, the Pacific Rim countries with the lowest death rates from prostate cancer also have the lowest fat consumption. In 1991, an American Cancer Society survey of 700,000 individuals demonstrated a correlation between obesity and clinical prostate cancer.

Cancer cells and normal cells

- Cancer Cells
- Normal Cells

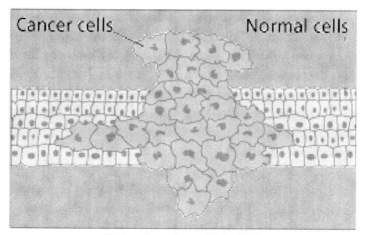
"Taken from CancerHelp UK"

Prostate cancer can be present for many years before it is discovered. In the earlier stages there are no symptoms, but as the cancer grows it can cause difficulties with urination, similar to those caused by BPH or prostatitis. If allowed to progress, the cancer can spread beyond the prostate. First it can spread to the lymph nodes and then to the bones of the hips and lower back, among others. Eventually it can spread to the lungs and more distant bones. Men may experience bone pain, weight loss, and fatigue when this occurs. Prostate cancer is often diagnosed during a routine physical when the physician performs a digital rectal exam (DRE) or a prostate specific antigen (PSA) blood test and finds a problem. There are four main tests doctors may use to detect problems in the prostate: feeling the prostate, a blood test, looking at the prostate with ultrasound, and biopsy.

DRE (Digital Rectal Examination): Still considered the "Gold Standard" of screening for prostate cancer, it is used to determine the prostate's general size, shape, and texture. For this test the physician inserts a gloved, lubricated finger into the patient's rectum and palpates the prostate through the rectal wall. This can be done quickly in the doctor's office with no preparation and is generally tolerated by most men. As a drawback, only the back surface of the prostate can be felt in this way; nothing can be examined about the front of the prostate. In the case of the very large prostate, a great deal of information is left out of the exam. The capsule of prostate is not well defined and can be difficult to identify in some areas, and it is not possible for doctors to determine if cancer has grown beyond the edge of the prostate. Accuracy of DRE also depends on the experience of the physician.

Rectal examination

- Rectum
- Physician places a gloved finger into your rectum and palpates the prostate through the rectal wall.

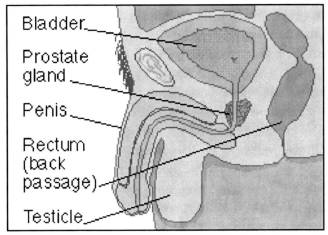

"Taken from CancerHelp UK"

Prostate Specific Antigen (PSA): This is a substance secreted by the prostate, and only the prostate, into the seminal fluid to dissolve the sperm clot after ejaculation. A small percentage of PSA leaks into the blood stream and is normally detectable in a blood sample. Many variables affect how much PSA ends up in the blood stream. In BPH, an enlarged prostate also makes PSA; therefore a man with BPH can have a higher, but still normal, PSA. Prostatitis can cause a rise in the level of PSA in the blood. Older men tend to have higher PSA levels, probably related to BPH. Prostate cancer cells produce ten times the amount of PSA as normal prostate cells.

A PSA level below four ng/ml is considered "normal," but there are no absolutes. More accurately speaking, the closer the value is to zero, the less likely the man is to have prostate cancer. The higher it is, and especially when the level rises above ten ng/ml, the more likely there is to be cancer. Change in the PSA level, tracked over time, can be a more accurate guide of what is happening. A steady upward climb in the PSA level, even if the value never gets above four ng/ml, can be an indicator of cancer. Acute prostatitis can cause a sudden jump in the PSA, but this will usually return to normal after the infection has cleared up. BPH can cause a high but stable level. Repeat or serial PSAs are useful in helping to differentiate between these diseases. The PSA is very sensitive to change in prostate, which makes it useful in addition to the DRE. Unfortunately, it is not specific to prostate cancer and requires experience to interpret the results. Screening symptomatic patients who do not demonstrate risk factors for prostate cancer with a PSA blood test is not recommended at this time in Canada by many doctors. However, many men choose to have this test, which is good. You and your doctor can discuss the risk factors, and you should make the decision whether it is appropriate for you. It should be your decision and not the doctor's. Men need to take more responsibility for their health and wellness; we have become too dependent.

Should the DRE or PSA show any abnormality, your doctor may recommend that you have a transrectal ultrasound of the prostate (TRUS) and a biopsy. Sound waves are used to create an image of the internal organs of the body. The prostate is viewed using a small probe placed in the rectum. The probe is covered with a condom and is well lubricated. It is no more uncomfortable or distasteful than having a DRE. Normally, you would be asked to take a small enema a few hours before the exam to ensure that the rectum is empty, but you are not usually required to fast. The exam only takes a few minutes.

Biopsies can be done through a guide attached to the ultrasound probe using a slender needle. You will be given an oral antibiotic to prevent any infection from occurring. There is not much feeling around the prostate, so discomfort is minimal. Generally no anesthetic is required, though sometimes a surface anesthetic gel may be used in the rectum. The physician performing the TRUS can very easily and accurately use biopsy to examine any lesions seen in the prostate. He or she may use the systematic samples through all parts of the prostate if nothing is seen or felt, but if the PSA looks suspicious, these samples will be examined by doctors specializing in pathology to determine whether or not there is cancer. Experts in assessing prostate cancer biopsies are available at specific labs and at certain medical centers.

The biopsy results will yield the Gleason grades. This is a subjective analysis by a pathologist of how the prostate cancer appears in the samples (biopsies) as compared to normal cells. The number will be between one and five for each Gleason grade, the higher number indicating a more aggressive cancer. The Gleason "score" or "sum" will be derived from adding the two grades. The first number indicates the predominant grade; the second number is the second most predominant grade. The predominant Gleason grade has to be at least 51 percent of the picture seen under the microscope. The secondary Gleason grade has to be at least 5 percent of the same picture. This is stated as, for example (3,3), which is the most common Gleason score. A Gleason score of (3,4) indicates that anywhere from 51 percent to 95 percent of the specimen is Gleason grade three disease and anywhere from 5 percent to 49 percent of the specimen has a secondary pattern of Gleason grade four disease. Gleason grade four and five disease are important negative prognostic indicators for the extent of disease and the clinical course of prostate cancer.

Samples can be sent to different expert pathologists for second opinions. Don't be afraid to ask for this additional assurance to make sure your Gleason score is correct, because this will be a major factor in your decision-making process. You should request a prostatic acid phosphatase (PAP) test after your diagnosis. This test can help determine if the cancer is most likely organ-confined or not. This blood test measures an enzyme in the blood. A PAP of 3.0 or higher is cause for concern. It is recommended that your PAP be sent to the same lab for consistency. Persistently elevated levels are considered possible evidence of metastases (spread of the cancer).

Prostascint is a relatively new technique in which a radioisotope is injected into the bloodstream. The isotope attaches itself to the cancer, and then a gamma camera is used to locate evidence of cancer if any is in your body. The test, like many of the others, is not 100 percent accurate, but it can be valuable in combination with other testing. The prostascint may indicate node involvement, in which case treatment options would be directed away from local therapy such as surgery, radiation, therapy, or oryotherapy.

Prostascint is used most often in the case of a recurrence of prostate cancer after local treatment of the gland, or in patients diagnosed with high-risk profiles for non-organ-confined prostatic cancer. The patient needs to be made aware that this test uses mouse antibodies. Some investigational clinical trials exclude anyone who has had prostascint test for this reason.

Endorectal MRI is used for establishing evidence of extracapsular extension. Particularly if it incorporates spectroscope, this technique is far superior to a routine pelvic MRI and is associated with a 75 percent to 90 percent accuracy rate when there is agreement between both modalities of imaging. This test is used to help determine the probability of organ-confined disease. This test is also useful in determining spread to seminal vesicles and regional nodes. It can also be extremely useful in detecting the site of prostate cancer in men suspected of having the disease but eluding diagnosis on routine ultrasound.

GUIDED BIOPSIES

Other tests such as DNA ploidy may be recommended to determine the nature of the cancer, its aggressiveness, and its responsiveness to androgen-deprivation therapies. Ploidy is a term used to describe the chromosome content of the cell population of a tumor. This would be particularly of interest to patients involved in hormone therapy and is used to determine the likelihood of the effectiveness of the treatment. Diploid cells have normal chromosome pairs and normal DNA. It is suggested by the physician's community that diploid cancer cells tend to grow slowly and respond well to hormone therapy. Aneuploid cancer cells have abnormal numbers of sets of chromosomes. Aneuploid cancer cells tend not to respond as well to hormone therapy and to be more aggressive. Aneuploid tumor are more often associated with high Gleason score prostate cancer (eight to ten) and non-organ-confined prostate cancer.

Bone scans are often done to determine if there is any evidence of metastases to the bone and should routinely be done if confirmed PSA is over ten. This is a precautionary measure and commonly done depending on your PSA and Gleason. It may come back negative or show signs of arthritis, in which case X-ray may be needed as confirmation. Be sure to tell your doctor of any past injuries to the bones that may show up as spots on the bone scan. You can discuss with your doctor the need for a bone scan if your PBA is ten or less and your Gleason score, validated by an expert, is six or less.

CT scan is another available tool depending on the results of other testing. If the cancer appears to be advanced, the CT scan determines what your treatment options are. Advanced prostate cancer is usually associated with PSA readings of fifty or higher and often Gleason scores of eight to ten. There is no guarantee that lower scores are not advanced. Some healthcare providers believe that CT scanning is a serious waste of healthcare dollars when used for tests on 90 percent of men with prostate cancer, because it is insensitive in detecting disease in the lymph nodes and valueless, in most patients, in detecting extra prostate extension such as capsular penetration or seminal vesicle involvement. In the setting of high PSA and/or high Gleason score, a CT scan may disclose lymph nodes that are greater than 1.0 centimeter in diameter. When such nodes are found they are associated with a specificity for prostate cancer of almost 100 percent.

CT scan could determine your treatment options.

- CT Scanning machine
- The couch that you lie on slides backward and forward
- The pictures are taken as you move through the machine

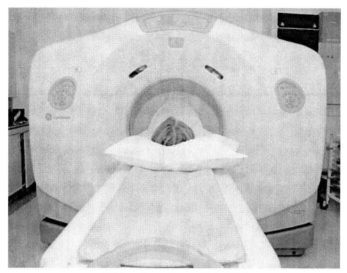
"Taken from CancerHelp UK"

CGA testing measure the blood levels of chromogramin A. This test is used to help identify patients with an aggressive form of prostate cancer and to help track their response to treatment. It is suggested that with progressive, and not just sporadically elevated, results CGA elevation in conjunction with elevations in other markers, such as NSE (neuron-specific enolase) or CEA (carcinoembyronic agent), is cause for serious concern of mutated aggressive prostate cancer. These findings should be put into context with the rest of the clinical and pathological pictures when making assessments. Do not allow yourself to be overwhelmed by them.

After the results of testing have been obtained, and prior to a treatment decision, you and your doctor should consult the parting tables to determine the probability of the disease confined in the organ or the probability of its spread to the seminal vesicles and the probability of the lymph node involvement. Healthy prostate cells are uniform in size and shape and are neatly arranged in the patterns of a normal gland. As cancer grows, they lose their healthy look. They change from normal well-differentiated tissues to more disorganized, poorly differentiated tissues. Eventually, a tumor develops.

Cancer cells

- Tumor is forming
- Cancer cells dividing

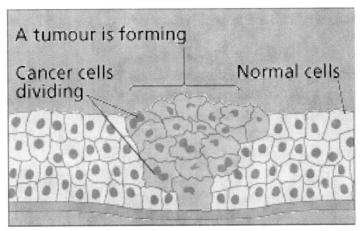

"Taken from CancerHelp UK"

Tumor grade is useful as a predictor of outcome. In one analysis, ten years after prostatectomy for localized cancer, prostate cancer had claimed the lives of 6 percent of the men whose cancer cells were well differentiated compared with 20 percent of those with moderately differentiated cancer cells and 23 percent of those with poorly differentiated cancer cells. The chances of developing metastatic prostate cancer followed a similar pattern. Ten years after surgery, metastasis was diagnosed in 13 percent of the men with well-differentiated tumors, but in 32 percent of those with cancers that were moderately differentiated and 48 percent of those whose cancers were poorly differentiated.

Cells that are completely differentiated know exactly what they are doing in life. Perfectly differentiated prostate cells are happy to go about their business in the prostate making PSA and ejaculatory juices. They look and act like the mature prostate cells they are. They interact with other perfectly differentiated prostate cells to create the tiny tubular structures that the prostate requires to deliver the product to the urethra. Once they become malignant, however, the prostate cells become less differentiated and behave less like well-disciplined prostate cells. The tubules they make with other malignant cells are distorted and haphazardly arranged. As they become even less differentiated, they form solid clumps and may become antisocial, preferring to go off on their own and not even attempt to make tubules with other cells.

Prostate cancer is staged using TNM system.

- T1 The tumor is too small to be seen
- T2 The tumor is in the prostate gland
- T3 The tumor has broken through the walls of the prostate
- T4 The tumor spread into other organs
- Stage T3 and T4 tumor are referred to as locally advanced prostate cancer

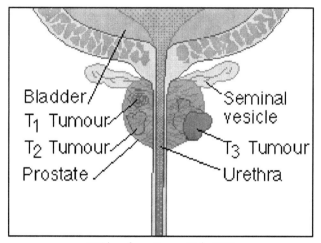

"Taken from CancerHelp UK"

When a certain type of cancer spreads to another part of the body, it does not change its type of cancer. For example, if a man with prostate cancer develops a tumor in the lung that is a metastasis from this prostate cancer, the tumor growing in the lung has the same characteristics as the prostate cancer. It does not represent a new lung cancer of the type that would develop if the cancer were to have started in or to be "primary" in the lung. Doctors believe this is important, because the treatment that will be effective against the metastasis will be the same treatment that will be used for the primary prostate cancer. This is why the doctors treating a patient think it is most important to establish the primary site at which any cancer originated.

Cancer can spread anywhere in the body. Some parts of the body are more vulnerable.

- Brain
- Skin
- Lung
- Lymph nodes
- Liver
- Bone

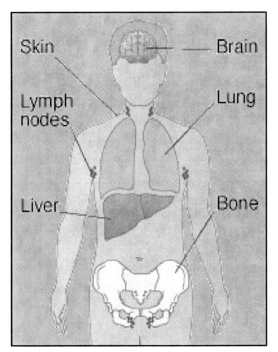

"Taken from CancerHelp UK"

Cancers do not spread in a completely random fashion. Some parts of the body are more vulnerable to becoming metastasis sites than others. For example, cancers metastasize to the skin, and they often metastasize to liver and lungs; also, each type of cancer has its own pattern for metastases. A very rare type of metastasis is caused by implantation or inoculation. This can happen accidentally when a biopsy is done or when cancer surgery is performed. In this case the malignant cells may actually drip from a needle or an instrument (this is also called a "spill").

It is suggested, therefore, that if possible and if the cancer is small, there is complete removal at the initial surgery of seminal vesicles to prevent the possibility of the cancer spreading into the lymph node.

Cancer leaves the prostate and spread to other organs.

- T4 Tumor invading other structures…

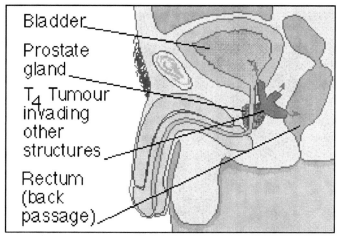

"Taken from CancerHelp UK"

Chapter 4:
Treatment of Prostate Cancer: The Conventional Methods

After all diagnostic tests are completed, your doctor can bring together all the information to make an educated guess about how much cancer is present and where it is located. This categorizing of the cancer helps to identify treatment choices that are best for each particular stage. When doctors talk about how much cancer is in a patient's body and exactly where it is located, they are referring to the stage of the cancer. The stage describes whether the cancer is small and confined to the prostate or large, with spread to any other tissues or organs, such as bones.

The stage is determined by information from the biopsies, the PSA level, the exam, and any additional tests and studies that may be done. The more cancer there is in your body, the more potential for spread and the less effective the treatments are likely to be. The more aggressive the cancers are as judged by the grade of the biopsy, the more likely the cancer will spread. Some physicians would consider a worse stage as reason to hold off on aggressive treatments, because the treatments probably won't be effective. Others argue that if there is an aggressive cancer, it is best approached with an aggressive treatment.

When the time comes to make decisions about cancer treatment, remember that you are in control. If you wish you can choose to let your doctor make the decisions, or you can retain control and use your doctor as a resource of information and opinions. Who actually decides what to do varies with each patient and his doctors. The usual scenario is for you to meet with your doctor so he can tell you what is wrong and what he wants you to do. The review of options is brief and often biased toward whatever he has decided is best for you.

Some physicians leave little time for your questions and concerns. Rarely are you encouraged to think about the various choices. A decision is almost always expected right then and there. In fact, sometimes the doctor goes so far as to schedule your treatment or surgery before you even arrive for your appointment. You must take an active role in deciding what you will do. For many years, doctors believed they knew what was best for patients. The doctor would proceed with the treatment without involving the patient and his family in decision making. Fortunately, those days are long gone. Today, the doctor's role is to gather information necessary to provide a fair and reasonable review of the facts and present a detailed discussion of the treatment options. The doctor should encourage you and your family to get involved in decisions. You are the one who will have to live with the outcome of the choice.

You are definitely the one who must decide which treatment is best for you. You can give this power to your doctor, but again this is your choice. Whether or not your doctor agrees with your decision, he/she should still be there to work with you and support your right to decide. Do not be alarmed if your doctor disapproves of your decision. Some doctors just aren't used to having someone disagree with them. Ask your doctor why he doesn't agree with your choice. He may have information that you had not considered, or a different approach. If your doctor will not respect your decision, you should find another doctor who will. There should be an open line of communication between you and your doctor; their opinion may be valid. Do not make your decision based on incomplete or inaccurate information.

There are about six basic treatment options offered by conventional medicine. They are as follows:

1) Simple watchful waiting, with monitoring of PSA level
2) Radical prostatectomy; abdominal or perineal
3) Radiation; external beam or radioactive seed plant
4) Hormone therapy; monthly injection or removal of the testicles
5) Cryotherapy; freezing the prostatic gland
6) Chemotherapy

Additionally there are a number of clinical trials and alternative options.

Watchful waiting: This is recommended for men believed to have early-stage cancer who are unlikely to feel its impact during their lifetime. This involves periodic visits to the urologist coupled with PSA testing to be sure that the prostate cancer continues to remain clinically insignificant.

Early-state prostate cancer offers a "window of curability," a period of time when a man has the best chance of being cured. The main trouble with watchful waiting is that it gives the cancer a chance to grow and spread beyond the prostate. If a man waits too long, the window of curability may shut forever. If you and your caregiver misjudge the situation—for example if the tumor was assigned too low a stage or grade—you will have fewer options available for containing the illness, and some of those options will pose serious risks. There are men who chose waiting rather than treatment for their early-stage cancer who have expressed regret at having missed the opportunity for a cure.

Radical Prostatectomy: Surgery is one of the common treatments of the prostate. A doctor may take out the cancer using one of the following operations: radical prostatectomy or transurethral resection. Radical prostatectomy is the removal of the prostate and some of the tissues around it, and also removal of the nearby lymph nodes. The doctor may do the surgery by cutting into the space between the scrotum and the anus. This operation is called a perineal prostatectomy. He/she may also do the surgery by cutting into the lower abdomen, which is called a retro-pubic prostatectomy. In many cases surgeons can remove the gland without cutting the nerves that control penile erection or bladder contraction, which makes such complications as impotence or incontinence less common than in the past.

Radical prostatectomy should only be done if the cancer has not spread outside the prostate, or if the patient is in good health. Age is also a factor. Often before the prostatectomy is done, the doctor will do surgery to take out lymph nodes in the pelvis to see if they contain cancer. This is called the pelvic lymph nodes dissection. If the lymph nodes contain cancer, usually the doctor will not do prostatectomy and may or may not recommend other therapy at this time.

Transurethral resection is a procedure in which the cancer is cut from the prostate using a tool with a small wire loop on the end that is put into the prostate through the urethra. This operation is sometimes done to relieve symptoms caused by the tumor, before other treatments, or in men who cannot have a radical prostatectomy because of age or other illness.

After surgery most men experience some degree of incontinence but may eventually regain complete urinary controls. It is difficult to say with confidence what percentage of men regain complete control, because there is no accurate survey. Impotence can also occur in most men treated by surgery. Doctors will tell you that post-op patients can manage impotence or incontinence resulting from surgery in a variety of ways. Impotence can be overcome with penile implants or other devices. Incontinence can be managed with special disposable underwear, condom catheters, or penile clamps. These are some of the results that scare many men from making critical decisions.

Radiation: Radiation therapy may be given as an alternative follow-up to surgery for cancer that has not spread. If cancer has spread to nearby tissue, radiation is the preferred treatment; it is also used in advanced cases to relieve pain from the spread of cancer to the bones. Radiation therapy or irradiation attempts to treat cancer by irradiating the cancerous cells to death, thus preventing them from growing and dividing. The idea is to kill off enough of the cancerous growth to shrink the growth, thereby making it less dangerous, reducing any pressure it might be placing on other parts of the body, and possibly reducing pain, bleeding, or other symptoms. However, be aware that radiation therapy does not cure cancer that has spread beyond the prostate. The two approaches used to deliver the radiation are external beam and internal seeds.

Radiation Machine

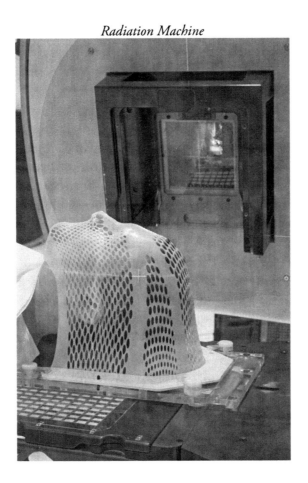

External beam radiation is what most people think of when they hear of "radiation." Some "radiologists" believe that radiation is as good as surgery for treating prostate cancer, with fewer side effects. (Surgeons of course, dispute these findings. They think that surgery is the best approach.) Radiation as mentioned above works by killing cells when they attempt to divide. If you take a biopsy of the prostate right after radiation, you will see cancer cells that seem to be intact. However, they can't divide and multiply, so they eventually die off. Radiation therapy typically begins by treating an area wider than the projected size of the cancer. The idea is that it's better to radiate a little too much and make sure that all the cancer is gone, rather than risk the regrowth of the cancer by letting even a few cells escape. The machine that delivers the radiation can be adjusted to "hit" the patient from various angles, including from below. Protective shields will be placed over other parts of the body for protection from the radiation. With radiation therapy, you can't be absolutely certain that the cancer has been completely eliminated.

Internal seed radiation, a method developed in the early 1970s, was called internal radiation, or radiation implants. Instead of hitting the patient with a radioactive beam, the doctors actually implanted little radioactive "seeds" inside the prostate. The idea was to get small doses of radiation exactly where it was needed, without having to pass through other parts of the body and without the risk of "overshooting" or missing the target. Cancerous cells near the implant die and are eliminated by the body. The early work with radiation implant was not successful, partially because doctors had to literally open the patient up in order to implant the radioactive seeds into the prostate. Then they had to "feel their way around" the prostate and guess as to the best spots for implanting the seeds or radiation in other areas.

Today the seeds are implanted through small needles pushed into the prostate via the perineum (the area between the scrotum and the rectum). Guided by images created by an ultrasound probe placed in the patient's rectum, the doctor inserts perhaps fifty to eighty seeds. This modern procedure is more accurate. Like surgery, good candidates for internal radiation seeds are men with early stages of cancers confined within the prostate and with PSA less than twenty and Gleason scores of seven or less.

Many men wish to avoid surgery, and for good reason. Despite the benefits of prostate surgery, it is not always the best solution. And even when surgery is indicated, some men are too frightened to agree to the procedure. Fortunately other therapies are available. From the understanding that the cancer cells growing in the prostate need testosterone to grow, some call testosterone the "fertilizer" for prostate cancer. Hormone therapy attacks prostate cancer by taking away testosterone.

Hormone therapy:Luteinising releasing hormone is triggered from the hypothalamus of the brain when our hypothalamus detects that decreasing levels of testosterone is received by receptors of the pituitary gland. This gland releases the luteinizing hormone. The hormone travels to the testicles to produce testosterone. In prostate cancer, hormone therapy, LHRH agonists and antagonists are medications that turn off the flow of testosterone from the testicles. Treatment consists of monthly injections. The process is that the hormone begins its work in the pituitary. The pituitary uses LHRH to stimulate the Leydig cells (cells inside the testes that stimulate testosterone). LHRH agonists interfere with the LHRH, making it impossible for the pituitary to signal the testes to produce testosterone. I will explain next the advantage of this procedure over surgery. The testicles are still in place, but they're not getting the "order" to make testosterone. The disadvantages have to do with costs and with the inconvenience of going back to your doctor's office once a month for injections.

Since most of the testosterone in a man's body is made by his testicles, as mentioned before, surgery is performed to remove the testicles in order to starve the cancer of testosterone. The surgical removal of one testicle is called an orchiectomy; removal of both is bilateral orchiectomy. Doctors describe this as a "minor procedure," but for the patient it is not that simple. The surgery is performed through an incision in the scrotum. The entire testis may be removed, or in a procedure called a subcapsular orchiectomy, it may be cored out and the outer shell left in place. It is a one-time procedure; you do not have to keep going back to the doctor's office for treatment once it is done. Given a choice, however, many men would prefer to keep their testicles. There are other procedures that I will not take time to discuss. However, when orchiectomy was the only form of hormone therapy available, it was reserved for only advanced cases. With the advent of new medication, however, hormone therapy is being used in early stages.

While hormone therapy is said to effectively halt the spread of cancer for some time, and even cause shrinkage of the tumor, prostate cancer cells eventually "learn" how to continue growing with only very little amounts of testosterone, or apparently without any at all. It may be that the cancer cells eventually become immune to the therapy, or perhaps the hormone therapy kills the bulk of the cancer cells, but those few that don't need testosterone multiply to the point at which they become dangerous once again. When that happens, hormone therapy is no longer effective. There is also the possibility that testosterone is not the hormone that influence cancer growth in the prostate.

Cancer cells do not obey signals they keep multiplying. Cancer cells keep doubling, regardless of the damage extra cells caused, to tissues and organs of the body. Cancer cells normally lose the molecules on their surface, that keep normal cells active and in the right place, at the right time. They become detached from there neighbors, and spread to other parts of the mind-body. Normal cells have special characteristics. They can reproduce, or stop reproducing at the exact time they are given a signal to stop. Normal cells, stick together in the right places, self district (apoptosis) if they are damage; become specialized or 'mature' in their duties. Cancer cells are the opposite. They keep reproducing, they do not obey signals from neighboring cells, they do not become specialized and they do not die. They move to other areas of the body and destroy normal cells. The body's healing systems must be involved in controlling and destroying cancer cells.

Cryotherapy: Cryotherapy is used to define several techniques in the medical community. The most common definition is the local or general use of low temperature in medical therapy. It is also called cryosurgery. It is a new and still relatively experimental technique where the prostate tissue is frozen. The purpose of this treatment is to kill the cancer cells. Doctors believe that this is a relative simple procedure; it is easy and quick and reduces cost. The quickness of cryosurgery is believed to make it potentially a better treatment than the prostatectomy or lengthy radiation treatments. Doctors at this point and time do not know if cryotherapy will be effective as a long-term treatment for prostate cancer. Cryosurgery is performed under anesthesia; special probes are placed throughout the prostate. Their positions are confirmed with rectal ultrasound. Liquid nitrogen is circulated through the probes, freezing the tissue of the prostate. A rectal ultrasound probe is used to monitor the freezing and to let the surgeon know when enough tissue has been treated. Their goal is to create an ice ball big enough to kill the cancer. According to supporters of this technique there is no damage to the adjacent bladder or to the rectal wall, which lies just behind the prostate. There are no long-term results to date, so supporters of this treatment don't know whether this will be as effective as radiation. The experts are presently hesitant to get too excited, because there are concerns that some cancer cells may escape being frozen and that others may be outside the prostate and cannot be treated.

Chemotherapy: Chemotherapy was essentially an investigational treatment. However, in the last thirty or more years, researchers have developed more anti-tumor drugs and supportive techniques that they suggest could reduce the side effects of the cancer-killing agents. They now believe that they have greater understanding of the nature of cancer and of how chemicals interact. With this understanding, chemotherapy has become a standard therapy. Chemotherapy is used alone or in combination with other treatments. Researchers and doctors have suggested that chemotherapy can cure some common forms of cancer.

However, there are a few things you should know about chemotherapy. First, it could affect your blood count. Chemotherapy often kills cells that are actively multiplying. Developing cells are multiplying continuously, as they mature in the bone marrow. These new cells are often killed by the chemotherapy drugs.

The white cell counts are affected first, because many white cells in the circulation system naturally die within a few days. Under normal circumstances, these cells are replaced by newly developed white cells. However, because these developing white cells are killed by chemotherapy, there will be a short wait before more new cells can be made. The process takes about a week or two. It may be just before your next course of chemo!

Mature red blood cells live for about three months. So you often don't get anemic or low in red cells until you're further into your chemotherapy course. Your doctor may want you to have a transfusion of red cells or a drug called erythropoietin, until your producing red cells are normal again.

Chemotherapy can also lower your platelet count. If that happens, you may get nose bleeds or a rash that looks like tiny bruises on your skin. Your doctor may recommend that you have a platelet transfusion. After a high dose of chemotherapy, it could take longer for the platelet count to get back to normal.

Brachytherapy: Brachytherapy is an outpatient technique that implants radioactive 'seeds' directly into the prostate. Implants can be temporary or permanent. Temporary implants are usually accompanied by external-beam radiation. This procedure requires more skill than external-beam radiation therapy, and with inexperienced physicians, the distribution of radioactive seeds is uneven in 15 percent of cases, increasing the risk for insufficient doses. It is suggested that computerized systems be developed to help oncologists optimize seed placement and allow precise treatment and higher radiation doses for each patient. Physicians hope that eventually, brachytherapy will improve the treatment of tumors, reduce side effects, and cut costs. Candidates selected and studied for this procedure are hoping that brachytherapy is useful, specifically those with prostate volumes less than sixty ml who have early-stage prostate cancer (T1 or T2 tumors, a Gleason grade lower than seven, and PSA levels below ten ng/ml). Doctors believe that it may also be beneficial in patients with inflammatory bowel disease or with cancer close to the bowel. Poor candidates for brachytherapy include men who have had TURP and patients with advanced cancer, high-grade tumors, or very enlarged prostate glands.

High Intensity Focused Ultrasound (HIFU): This is a technique using focused ultrasound to generate areas of intense heat to destroy tissue in the prostate. It has been promoted as noninvasive therapy for localized prostate cancer. It is also used for tumor of liver and other sites. It is suggested that in its ten years existence, thousands of men have been treated with HIFU. Most patients have been treated in Europe. The National Institute for Clinical Excellence, a government body in the United Kingdom which evaluates new treatments, has reviewed the clinical data and concluded that the evidence is sufficient and recommended its use within the UK's National Health System. HIFU is not new to North America; however, it is not approved by the United States' FDA. The procedure is available in Canada. It is promoted as experimental by independent authorities. Ultrasound has been used for medical imaging for many years, but recently the technology has been developed so that it can be used for treatment as well as diagnosis all types of cancer and other tissue diseases.

For many years, researchers have been looking for one single drug, a "magic bullet" that could cure cancer. This drug has not been found; however, there are a few new biological drugs that specifically target certain cancers. There are about fifty or more biological anticancer drugs available on the market. Some have not been approved for general distribution but have been used to treat some form of cancer. These experimental or investigational drugs are supplied to clinical trial investigators under a special government license. To make drugs available earlier for therapy, some drugs that are believed to have an established role in treatment are made available to practicing oncologists, even though they are not yet on the retail market. Once again the responsibility lies with the person who is sick to make the final decision.

Chapter 5:
Living with Side Effects Caused by Conventional Treatments

Dealing with the serious side effects of prostate problems can be very stressful for men and their families; therefore every man who must make a decision regarding his prostate cancer should talk to another man who has had the disease. Doctors and books can give you all kinds of information and statistics, but only a man who has been there can tell you what it's like to go under the knife, to be radiated, or to refuse treatment. Only a man whose nerve bundles have been damaged can tell you what it's like to temporarily or permanently lose the ability to have an erection; only a man who has lost the ability to hold his urine can give you his experience. Talking and listening to men as they open up at prostate support groups, and reading their stories, is an educational experience for me. Some of the stories are sad, some are humorous, some are frightening, and some are inspirational.

Urinary incontinence, the inability to hold your urine, is one of the side effects of prostate cancer treatment. The muscles at the base of the bladder and right below the prostate help men to control their urine. Unfortunately, surgery and radiation can damage this urinary-control mechanism. Other problems can cause incontinence, including a damaging growth left untouched by the surgeon's knife, urethral strictures, urinary tract infections, and some medicines.

Eliminating your urine is important, but inability to hold your urine is a problem.

All the organs below are important in the urine-nary system.

- Your kidneys
- Ureter
- Bladder
- Prostrate
- Urethra

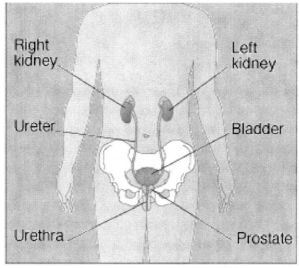

"Taken from CancerHelp UK"

We do not know exactly how many men with prostate problems develop incontinence, because the estimates vary considerably from study to study. It is suggested that the incontinence rate following radical prostatectomy is very high. Estimates in urological literature vary widely, with some researchers stating that only 2.5 percent of men become incontinent and others saying that the actual incidence is well over 80 percent. Beside the messy inconvenience, incontinence following prostatectomy may also be psychologically devastating for men who had no urinary problem before surgery. Eventually some men can learn how to use the muscles damaged during surgery. Men are strongly encouraged to begin Kegel exercises even before surgery.

There are about three types of incontinence; however, the results are the same. There is stress incontinence, losing urine when sneezing, laughing, or coughing, or when moving in certain ways. Men with stress incontinence may leak urine when they get off a chair, get out of bed, or move about, exercise, or walk.

Urge incontinence is losing urine as soon as the urge hits before one can get to the bathroom. Some men may have to go after drinking even small amounts of liquid. Overflow incontinence is feeling that the bladder is never really empty. Men with overflow incontinence often dribble urine throughout the day and night, spend a lot of time in the bathroom, pass only small amounts of urine at a time, and have a dribble rather than a flow.

Your doctor may use blood tests, urinalysis, or urodynamic testing if you complain of incontinence. A post-void residual measurement (PVR) may also be recommended, which involves using ultrasound and a small tube placed in the bladder to measure how much urine remains in your bladder after you urinate. A stress test may also be used to see how much urine you lose when exercising, coughing, or performing other tasks.

Treatment depends on the type of incontinence. Once this has been established, treatment may begin, including such nonmedical, nonsurgical methods as bladder training and exercise for the pelvic muscles. Bladder training is useful for urge and stress incontinence. Exercises for the pelvic muscles, called Kegel exercises, help strengthen weakened muscles around the bladder. You will be reminded by your doctor to squeeze your outlet muscle before standing up, before bending, squatting, lifting, or before doing anything else that may cause leakage.

Medications are used to help eliminate infections that cause urinary problems, to stop abnormal contractions of the bladder muscles, and to tighten up weakened sphincter muscles. Drugs used include Propantheline, Bromide, Flavoxate, Phenylpropanolamine, and Pseudoephedrine. Unfortunately, all drugs have some side effects, and taking additional drugs to relieve the problem cause by previous treatment can add stress, frustration, and sometimes depression.

Surgical treatments are applied where portions of the prostate gland may be pressing against the bladder or prostatic urethra and can be cut away and weak pelvic muscles can be reinforced or supported. There are many surgeries doctors use to relieve incontinence, depending upon the cause of the problem. Surgeons can even implant artificial sphincters. Surgeries are risky because they involve cutting into the body, and once surgeries have been performed they cannot easily be undone, especially if something has been removed. There is healing that works by giving yourself time. In a fair number of men, urinary control will gradually reappear in the months following surgery as damaged nerves apparently repair themselves. One should make pelvic muscle exercise a part of his daily routine.

All aspects of prostate cancer and treatments can somehow have an impact on erections. Surgery and radiation can damage the nerves and blood vessels that allow men to achieve and maintain erections. Hormone therapy can often eliminate erection through unknown mechanisms. In addition, lack of interest can sometimes accompany the loss of testosterone. It is suggested that 24 to 40 percent of men who undergo radiation therapy will become impotent. Unlike surgery, where impotence is immediate, radiation may cause problems that may occur slowly. Even if the man has had great erections before or even during and after radiation treatments, many men still describe a slow loss of erections over about one year's time. It is believed to be a result of radiation injury to the small blood vessels and nerves.

After interstitial seed therapy up to 65 percent of men who had good erections before treatment will have significant problems with erection afterward. Like external-beam therapy, in seed therapy it can take quite a while before loss of erections is manifested.

With radical surgery there is the potential for the tiny nerves that transmit messages that cause an erection to be cut or damaged when removing the prostate. If the message can't get to the penis to allow blood in, there will be no erections. In addition there may be injury to the blood supply that helps with erections. However, in the last several years a modification of the radical prostatectomy procedure has been developed that spares the nerves that control erection. These nerves run very close to the prostate gland in small bundles on either side of the prostate.

It is suggested by physicians that when the nerve-sparing operative procedure is done successfully, erectile functions remain good in the majority of patients. However, there are urologists who are concerned that by sparing the nerves controlling erection the efficiency of the operation may be compromised, because in order to spare the nerves it is necessary to "shave" the margins of the prostate gland quite closely, so that if the cancer goes right up to the true capsule of the prostate and perhaps through it, there is the possibility of leaving cancer behind in the patient. It appears that nerves can often be damaged when the prostate is frozen, resulting in erectile dysfunction in up to 80 percent of men. As with surgery, there is a fine line between trying to kill all the cancer with freezing and preserving nerve function. The procedure is not precise enough to tell exactly where to stop the freezing process so that all the cancer is killed and yet the nerves are left undamaged.

The male hormone is responsible for much of the male sex drive called libido. In addition, testosterone plays an important role in the ability to get an erection. When testosterone is eliminated from the body, it is common for men to become impotent. A loss of muscle mass and fatigue are common. Many men also experience hot flashes, and some suffer gastrointestinal symptoms. There are medicines to deal with hot flashes and gastrointestinal symptoms, and there are treatments for impotence. However, these treatments come with side effects also. Whereas some men are able to continue enjoying sexual intercourse during hormonal therapy, others are psychologically devastated by the loss of their manhood.

There is also physical, mental, and emotional pain caused by all the side effects that can last for a lifetime. Many of these treatments may only halt the spread of cancer for some time or even cause shrinkage of the tumor. Prostate cancer cells eventually continue to grow in some men after all the stressful therapy they undergo. It may be that the cancer cells eventually become immune to the therapy and become more dangerous once again. When this happens treatment is no longer effective. Unfortunately, regardless of the treatment, a certain number of men will suffer from an inability to have an erection depending on the type of therapy used. As many as 50 to 60 percent of men will suffer from at least short-term impotence. For many it will be permanent.

There are some techniques used for helping men with impotence. One is injection of a substance called PEG directly into the base of the penis, using a fine needle. This procedure produces satisfactory erections in most men. One of the dangers with the injections is priapism, a condition in which the penis continues to remain hard for hours. Such a man will need to seek medical help if the erection last for three to four hours to prevent serious injury or gangrene of the penis. There are also tissue scars caused by the injections.

Other devices for helping men with impotence are vacuum devices and implants. There are several different styles of implants, but they work on the same principles. The devices are long thin tubes that are surgically implanted into the spongy part of the penis on the underside and on each side of the urethral tube. Some complications resulting from the use of these devices include infections, narrowing of the urethra, and deformities of the penis. Many of the devices have had to be removed, often resulting in shrinkage of the penis.

Learning that you have cancer is a powerful blow to almost every man. But what you do after getting the news is important. Most men go along with their doctor's recommendations, placing their lives most times in the hands of strangers. For a while they may feel that they have no control over their lives as they submit to rounds of tests and consultations, then to treatment and its aftermath. Other men prefer to look upon their cancer as a challenge. Determined to stay in control of their lives, they insist upon choosing their own treatment. Those men who decide to fight the disease (those who look upon the disease as a challenge) tend to do better than those who surrender.

Men's emotional responses to an opinion of their treatments vary. Some men are pleased; others are dissatisfied and angry. Even when the therapy seems to go well, some men are unhappy, while others take their troubles in stride. However, most men are more concerned with impotence and incontinence.

Quotes from a Few Survivors

"I have been put in a prison of positivity by a society that expects things to go back to normal when you are cured or in remission. The doctors are so caught up in treating disease that they forget that it is housed in a person! My aim is to bring about a change in the approach of the medical professions by forcing them to treat the mind of the patient and primary care/partner by constantly checking on how the disease and treatment is affecting their well-being. Society also needs to be taught how to treat both patients and new survivors—we cannot act as if nothing has happened. Our lives are permanently altered and often a new outlook and attitude arises. My whole stage of illness and treatment left me suicidal and without any support from my wife and those I expected to care. I am now getting a divorce and am focused on friends who care for me now, my family and anyone touched by cancer who is lost in the whirlpool of the treatment cycle. I am trying to set up an advocacy group of survivors to help speak for those who are too ill or confused to know where to turn for advice." survivor." M.P.

"Hello, my name is Bob and I am a testicular cancer survivor. I had my cancerous testicle removed in November of 91 and then a Lymph Node Dissection due to the cancer spreading, then six weeks of intensive chemotherapy I am 100 percent cancer-free and also the proud father of a one-year-old baby girl. If anyone needs to talk or is experiencing testicular cancer, please feel free to write." Good Luck and God Bless, Robert J.

"In 1990, I went to the doctor and he determined that my prostate was, oh, five times as big as it should be. The only symptom I had was that I went to urinate; it was very bloody. The doctor decided to do a PSA and a biopsy. It was negative. After that, I had a PSA every six months, and I had a total of three biopsies, all were negative but my PSA was slowly creeping up from

eight to nine. Finally, in 1994 the doctor said, 'Let's do another biopsy. And this time I'm going to do four on each side.' Sure enough, they came back positive. He said the cancer might have been there before, but I don't see how he could have missed it with the previous three biopsies. The way the doctor explained it to me, there's only one cure for prostate cancer. If it hasn't escaped the prostate, take it out. I had the surgery a month ago, and I've only had the catheter out for two weeks. My control is already coming back, especially at nights. I've been working on my exercises."

"How about the sexual complication?" "We sat down and talked about it and the doctor explained the different methods I could try after surgery. When I'm ready, I am going to try the injection method. I don't see why the impotence won't improve as quickly as the incontinence did."

"Knowing what you now know would you go back and change your treatment if you could?" "No I would have done the same thing, even if the cancer had spread."

"Do you have any advice for a man who has just learned that he has prostate cancer?" "You've got to have a positive mental attitude. As soon as they let me know I had prostate cancer, I went to a support group. And I immediately started doing visualization on killing the cancer cells, keeping them contained in the prostate." Jerry

"I didn't have any symptoms, but at a regular check up the doctor found that there was something wrong when he did the finger/rectal examination. My PSA was 38. The urologist told me that I had to have a biopsy and when I did, he told me that I had to have surgery."

"Did the doctor explain all the options to you?" "Yes, he did. But the way he explained the options, there were no options."

"Do you feel that the doctor's explanation was slanted in favour of surgery?" "Yes. The doctor didn't explain nearly enough for me to fully understand what was going to happen."

"Are you sorry that you had the surgery?" *"I regret having the surgery. It turned my life upside down."*

"Why is that?" *"They cut the nerve to my penis when they cut out my prostate. Physically, I can't have sexual relations because I can't have an erection. I have to give myself an injection to do anything. I have a problem with leaking. If I sneeze or cough, I leak. If I try to lift something, my pants get wet. It's depressing; it's embarrassing. It is all psychologically very painful. With the urine problem and the sex problem, I'm depressed to the point that I just don't want to stay alive anymore. I wish they had just cut off my penis and testicles; then I would be done with it entirely."* Alvin.

The diagnosis of cancer can be a turning point in many people's lives. The fear of death or in some cases the knowledge that death is imminent has a remarkable way of focusing and clarifying one's thoughts. For some people, the diagnosis is a devastating experience. For others, it's a call for action. For some people the diagnosis is a call to evaluate relationships with family, friends, relatives, and God.

Prostate cancer is a "couple's disease." It not only affects the man, but his sexual partner and his family, his loved ones. Stress and depression are common consequences of dealing with the diagnosis, the treatment decision, the treatment itself, and the side effects of the treatment. If depression becomes severe and overwhelming, it is appropriate to seek professional help. People deal with life cases in their own ways. It is especially important to be good to yourself and the people whom you care about and who care about you and will give you the strength to overcome the disease. From those of us who have been there, the recommendation is to try to move beyond the panic with knowledge because knowledge is power. You should do your research and arrive at the best treatment decision for you and your family, based on the characteristics of your own health situation.

An article on prostate treatment in the *Boston Globe* on January 18, 2003, by Ann Barnard titled "The Truth" stated that a robust fifty-six-year-old man who faced surgery for prostate cancer was terrified that it would leave him impotent. He made the rounds, visiting top urologists at Harvard hospitals. He chose a surgeon who told him that 80 percent of his patients end up able to have sex without the help of devices. Last week, unable to get an erection and suffering from incontinence, he went to a support group at Beth Israel Deaconess Medical Center, where he learned that the vast majority of the group had significant trouble with sexual function, even years after surgery or radiation treatment. It turns out that the 80 percent success rate may be more hope than reality, achieved only by few highly practiced surgeons on selected patients. One large-scale study of prostate cancer survivors found that eighteen months after treatment, 60 percent could not get an erection firm enough for intercourse. As a result, men, including some in the Beth Israel support group, feel they were misled about the sexual side effects of their treatment.

"Why can't we get good solid information?" Asked the Boston man at Beth Israel, who at four months after surgery still hopes for improvement and did not want his name used for fear of alienating his doctor.

If people knew the truth, if there were more information given by doctors regarding side effects and other implications, I think people could deal with this disease a little better. Doctors agree that there is a broad gap between the more optimistic potency rates widely quoted in surgeons' books and Web sites—especially those of celebrity specialists like Johns Hopkins Hospital's Dr. Patrick C. Walsh—and the more typically experienced doctors. Published studies report post-surgical rates of impotence ranging from less than 15 percent to more than 80 percent, depending on the patient's age and condition and the experience of the surgeon.

Radiation treatment offers a somewhat lower risk of impotence, but because long-term survival is not so good, doctors usually recommend surgery for younger patients, the ones most likely to be sexually active. However, doctors say they tell patients up front about risks and tradeoffs. They also say that support groups overstate the degree of dissatisfaction because they tend to attract more men who are having problems to their group. But some doctors, as well as many patients, believe that the prostate cancer survivors have a point: Surgeons sometimes downplay the chances of impotence as they focus on curing cancer. They sometimes quote potency rates for celebrity surgeons who do nothing but remove prostates, rather than their own rates, said Dr. Jeffrey Steinberg, acting chief of surgery at Cambridge Health Alliance, who advises the support groups of younger, healthier patients.

The result, said group leader Stan Klein, is that with 180,000 men diagnosed and 55,000 undergoing prostate removal surgeries each year, thousands of survivors are glad to be alive, but painfully disappointed with their sexual function.

The reality of life after prostate cancer treatment is highly underestimated by many conventional healthcare-treatment providers. They publicly speak for men whose lives they do not understand. Only a man who has experienced the physical, mental, and emotional pain, and sometimes lifelong suffering, can understand the need and support many men require. How can a doctor understand the feelings of a man who lies beside his wife night after night hoping and wishing that things were normal, that just for one moment he could have an erection? This is reality, not fiction. I have a friend who had surgery for prostate cancer; his mother told me that he is having serous incontinence problem and he does not want to talk to anyone about it. She asked me to give him a call, but I should not mention his problem. She was hoping that talking to me and knowing that I had surgery for prostate cancer would give him the opportunity to talk about his problem. I have spoken to him several times, and to date he has not mentioned his surgery for prostate cancer.

Many men are living in seclusion and denial. They are pretending that they are living a normal life and everything is okay, but on the inside they are crying for help. Some men are blessed by having loving wives and family members to provide support in their time of need. There are many men who may have lost their wives or lady friends because of the side effects from prostate cancer treatment. What is so sad about all this is that many of the healthcare providers and government food and drug administrators spend more time and money fighting over treatment procedure and status. In my research I have read so many articles describing healthcare providers as quacks because they believe in natural therapies, and some alternative healthcare providers are fighting back by discrediting all conventional treatment. All of this fighting is taking centre stage, while there is so much mental, physical, and emotional pain and suffering affecting the lives of many men and their families.

"The relationship that exists between the mind and body is very intimate. When one is affected, the other sympathizes. The condition of the mind affects the health to a far greater degree than many realize. Many of the diseases from which men suffer are a result of mental depression. Grief, anxiety, discontent, remorse guilt, distrust, all tend to break down the life forces and to invite decay and death."

It is suggested by psychologists that we are only beginning to understand the connection between disease and the mind. There is a fast-growing group of researchers studying the relationship between emotion, personality, characteristics, and disease, especially cancer. Several psychological characteristics appear to influence the course of cancer: depression, anxiety, lacking a sense of control, having a negative outlook, and lacking added support system to sustain stability.

A study has shown that people who have characteristics and the ability to express emotion and fight against cancer influence the outcome of the disease. Chronic depression has been identified as an element in the development of cancer. In 1975 Dr. Steven Greer and Tina Morris reported that women with malignant breast tumors had more difficulty in expressing anger than those with benign tumors. Greer also found that cancer patients who had a fighting spirit lived longer than those who felt helpless or hopeless.

These studies are showing us that patients' wills to live or fighting spirits have a great deal to do with their chances for a recovery. Emotions, either positive or negative, influence our ability to survive in an environment of high stressors. "Stress is not from without; it is from within." Those who are engage in a positive outlook save energy and give their mind/body a better chance to fight the disease. While negative emotions predict a poorer prognosis for cancer patients, positive feelings such as joy, peace, and tranquility go together with a better outcome. A seven-year follow-up study of breast cancer patients by Sandra Levy, associate professor of psychiatry and medicine in oncology at the Pittsburgh Cancer Institute, showed that those patients who expressed more joy in their lives when initially tested live longer. "Courage, hope, faith, sympathy, love, promote health and prolong life. A contented mind, a cheerful spirit, is health to the body and strength to the soul."

When I was preparing to undergo surgery for prostate cancer, I met a young lady at the blood bank. She looked so healthy and full of life. She told me she had surgery for liver cancer five years before, and the cancer came back. She happily suggested that after her next surgery, she hope to live another five years. There was no pessimism, remorse, or hopelessness in her attitude. I hope she is still alive. In contrast I met another young lady in the hospital after I had surgery. She also had surgery for liver cancer, and she was very pessimistic—she told me that she was going to die. She went home, and I kept in touch with her husband. She died two month after leaving the hospital. I was not surprised, because she had no will to live. Bernie Siegel told of one of his patients: As soon as she was diagnosed with having cancer she went home and donated her clothes to Goodwill Industries. This act demonstrated that she believed the disease would eventually kill her, so she might as well give up.

The attitudes people have when they discover that they have cancer range from determination to fight the disease to denial to utter hopelessness and despair. A highly significant study published in 1979 showed that cancer patients who were rated as less cooperative by doctors and nurses lived longer. The research also suggested that more difficult patients receive less radiotherapy. This could be attributed to the patients taking more control over their treatment and their lives. Thus they chose more appropriate levels of treatment, which elevated their self-esteem. In general those patients who are determined to take control of their own therapy and destiny are the most likely to get well, and those are not seen as good patients by doctor.

Healthcare providers should put themselves in the place of men who are suffering from prostate cancer and the side effects caused by treatments. Most of these men don't have any prejudice against any form of treatment; their greatest aspiration is to get well. They don't worry about the process; their main concern is the result. It takes great wisdom and compassion to deal with these men who may be depressed and weak from fear of the unknown. Because of these facts, healthcare providers have the moral and ethical obligation to provide their patient or client with facts. Physicians owe it to themselves and their patients to become at least familiar with the more commonly used herbal products and natural treatments and to decide whether and how to integrate them into their practices. Honesty in dealing with a patient inspires him with confidence and provides an important pathway to recovery.

In my research, I was overwhelmed and sometime sad to read of the hundreds of so-called cures and treatments for prostate and other cancer. Every week there is discovery of a new drug or new product to cure prostate and other cancer. The media overkill influences many men in their decision making. It would make a difference if more time and money were spent on education about lifestyle changes, nutrition, and prevention.

Chapter 6:
An Alternative Approach to Prevention and Treatment

The alternative approach to the management and treatment of the prostate and prostate cancer is quite different from the conventional approach and perhaps more beneficial for some men. I am not necessarily recommending any of these therapies. The information on alternative treatment and prevention is for information only. Whenever a man is experiencing symptoms with his urinary system, he should check with his doctor.

A fascinating study released in 1993 showed that Americans have a great deal of faith in alternative medicine. On the other hand, perhaps the study shows that they are losing faith in standard Western medicine. Whatever the reason, people are turning to alternative forms of healing in greater numbers than ever before, and they are spending more money out-of-pocket for traditional medicine. Perhaps part of the appeal of alternative therapies is that, for the most part, they are not nearly as toxic or potentially dangerous as are the powerful drugs, radiation, chemotherapy, surgeries, hormone therapy, and other conventional treatment.

Prolactin: Prolactin is a hormone that encourages the prostate to take in more testosterone and convert it to DHT. It is the DHT that stimulates the prostatic overgrowth of BPH. Some researchers feel that an ingredient (or a combination of ingredients) found in beer stimulates the pituitary gland to release more prolactin. Thus, avoiding beer has been proposed as a simple, nontoxic way of realigning body chemistry and reducing the symptoms of BPH.

Hydrotherapy: The ancient treatment called hydrotherapy is the use of hot water, cold water, ice, or steam to treat disease and improve overall health. Because of its physical properties related to conditions of heat, buoyancy, and cleansing action, water is an ideal agent for applications of heat and cold to obtain desired physiological effects, debridement of wounds that are extensive and not easily cleansed by other methods, and the implementation of programs of therapeutic exercise. Application of cold and warm water help relieve pain and improve circulation, promote relaxation and reduce muscle tightness, and serve to localize infections. In the treatment of BPH, patients use a small tub called a sitz bath, in which the buttock and lower belly are immersed in water. A warm bath (up to 99° F) is used for acute prostatitis; a hot bath (up to 115°F) is used to open urinary passageways for patients with nonacute prostatitis; and a cold bath (between 55° F and 75° F) following a warm or hot bath is used for general health benefits once the prostate problem has been cured. Contrast baths, with alternating hot and cold water, may be used to improve muscle tone and circulation in the pelvic area.

Plant products have been found to be helpful in reducing prostate swelling, alleviating the pain, and reducing certain other symptoms. These natural health aids include prostat, pygeum africanum, Equisetum arvense, hydrangea, arborescens, serenoa serrulata, and saw palmetto. Hydrangea root diuretic helps prevent stones or gravel. It helps to dissolve hard deposits in the veins and urinary system. It's also used in the treatment of inflamed or enlarged prostate glands, and is helpful with urinary stones. Aloe arborescens extracts have been investigated and shown to have wound-healing, anti-bacterial, anti-ulcer, anti-inflammatory, anti-carcinogenic, hypoglycemic properties.

Prostat: Prostat contains an extract from pollen that has been used to treat BPH in Europe and Japan for years. In European studies of chronic prostatitis, 78 percent of men have had a favourable response to prostat alone. Prostates enlarge when testosterone is converted into DHT within the prostate. Prostat shrinks the prostate by occupying the DHT receptors and locking out testosterone; thus DHT cannot be made and the prostate shrinks. The man's overall testosterone supply is left undisturbed; only the testosterone by-product in the prostate is affected. European and American studies are quite promising: Prostat relieves some of the symptoms of prostate problems and shrinks the enlarged prostate. It is nontoxic and seems to be well tolerated. A study reported in the *British Journal of Urology* compared a prostat called Cernilton in Europe to a placebo in a double-blind study of sixty men with urinary difficulties due to BPH. Following the six-month study, the authors concluded that prostat has a beneficial effect in BPH and may have a place in the treatment of patients with mild or moderate symptom of overflow obstruction. Another study looked at the effects of the pollen extract on ninety men ages nineteen to ninety suffering from prostatitis and prostatodynia. The researchers found it to be "effective in the treatment of patients with chronic nonbacterial Prostatitis and Prostatodynia." However, it did not help those with complicating factors, such as strictures in the urethra or calcification of the prostate.

Pygeum Africanum: This product of all African evergreen trees has a long history of use for urinary tract difficulties. Although only recently available in United States, it has been studied for over twenty years. Controlled, double-blind studies have shown pygeum to be very helpful in reducing prostate inflammation and symptoms of prostatitis. It has been used for prostate problems in Europe for some time. Researchers have also noted that Equisetum helps to reduce prostatic inflammation and its attendant symptoms.

Serenoa Serrulata: Berries of the American dwarf palm were part of the regular diet for some American Indians. In the nineteenth century, serenoa was noted for its toning affects on the male reproductive system. It is felt that serenoa blocks the formation of dihydrotestosterone (DHT) as well as the ability of DHT to bind to receptor cells in the prostate. Serenoa has been shown to increase urinary flow rate and to reduce the mean residual volume (what is left in the bladder after urination).

Saw Palmetto: Saw palmetto is extracted from a palm tree native to the Atlantic coast and the West Indies and has long been used to rejuvenate prostate problems. It is felt that saw palmetto's beneficial effects on prostate are due to its ability to inhibit DHT, thus helping to keep the prostate at the normal size.

Reflexology: Reflexology treats ailments by massaging certain areas of feet or hands. This art goes back at least 5,000 years to the Chinese, and it was used by some Egyptians as far back as 3,000 B.C. According to reflexologists, the body is divided into many zones running up and down or across the body. The kidney is treated, for example, by locating it with the "gridwork," then treating (massaging) the corresponding area on the feet and hands. Although no one knows exactly why reflexology works, some of the theories that have been advanced for the success of the therapy include the following: It improves blood circulation; it stimulates the nervous system; it realigns energy system within the body; it stimulates acupuncture points; it encourages the drainage of lymph fluid; and it removes crystal deposits of calcium at the end of the nerves in the feet. Overall the attempt in reflexology is to balance the body, helping it to heal itself.

To treat prostate problems associated with infection and enlargement, the reflexologist will massage foot points corresponding to the prostate, the pituitary gland, the thyroid gland, the adrenal glands, the lymph system, the urethras, and the kidneys. The foot points corresponding to the urinary system are found on the bottom half of the right sole, on the foot. In the hand the prostate point is slightly below the thumb, on the edge of the hand.

Ayurveda medicine: Ayurveda medicine is an ancient medical system from India based on the principle that the mind and body are one, so the body cannot be well if the mind is troubled. Only recently introduced to the United States, Ayurveda is a holistic healing system that uses diet, massage, detoxification, herbal remedies, and breathing exercises to treat ailments. According to Ayurveda philosophy, there are many possible causes of cancer itself resulting from physical, emotional, and spiritual imbalances. The three-stage treatment for cancer attempts to detoxify, balance, and rebuild the body through diet, herbs, meditation, spiritual and emotional therapy, and cleansing. Yoga, the chanting of mantras, and gem therapy may also used to enhance the body's aura.

Homeopathy: Homeopathy was developed in the late 1700s by Samuel Hahnemann, a German physician. Unlike in standard Western medicine, practitioners of homeopathy believe that "like cures like." In other words a person with disease A can be cured by being administered a tiny dose of a substance that causes the symptoms of disease A in a healthy person. This principle is very similar to that underlying vaccine (a little bit of a germ helps the immune system fight off a full-fledged invasion of the same germ). Whereas standard medicine looks upon symptoms as terrible things to be stamped out, homeopathy views symptoms as proper adaptations of the body to problems. Symptoms come about because the body is trying to heal itself. Thus, instead of using powerful drugs to eliminate the symptoms, homeopathy attempts to help the body heal itself. The homeopathic doctor will use a small dose of a highly diluted homeopathic medicine to stimulate the body's natural healing processes.

The homeopath expects symptoms to be cured in the reverse order in which they appeared, and possibly to get worse before they get better. However, the patient should feel better overall, because the body is stronger. Here are some of the homeopathic medicines that might be used for prostatitis (inflammation of the prostate): Staphysagria, for urinary streams that stop and start and for burning; Pulsatilla, for pain after urinating and for penile discharges; Kalibichromicum, for severe prostate pain worsened by movement, burning after urination, and certain penile discharges; Caustieum, for urinary leakage when coughing, sneezing, or laughing, for pain following urination, and for retention of urine following surgery; Sabal serrulata, for frequent urination and pain in the perineal area. There are other homeopathic medicines that may be given two to three times daily for several days and then stopped as soon as the symptoms improve. The medicines are given one at a time, not in a group.

Oriental Medicine: According to the theory of Oriental medicine, prostatitis is caused by weakness or other difficulties in the kidney, spleen, or liver meridians. There are twelve meridians, or invisible energy pathways, in the body. Prostate problems may be caused by weakness in the kidney meridians, by dampness in the spleen meridian, by a blockage in the liver meridian, or by any combination of the three. According to Oriental medicine, all prostate conditions ranging from an infection to cancer are due to problems with one or more of the three pertinent meridians. A greater problem with the meridians means a more severe illness. Thus, all treatment aims to build up the kidney meridian, dry up the dampness in the spleen meridian, and/ or remove the blockage in the liver meridian. The more severe the problem, the stronger, more stringent, or longer the treatment, but the basic principle will remain the same unless there is an actual growth (such as a tumor), which will then require specific herbs to break it up. There are genetic dietary, emotional, and other factors contributing to problems with the meridians. The kidney meridian, for example, may be weakened through a lifetime of stress. The liver meridian may be harmed if one is an alcoholic. The treatment for the prostate problem is highly individual, and it depends upon the individual's specific problems, overall health, and the type of doctor consulted or Oriental medicine used. In general, however, treatment consists of acupuncture, Chinese herbal combinations, emotional changes, and diet to eliminate problems with the affected meridians.

Detoxification Therapies: Detoxification therapies use safe and effective detoxification methods to alleviate from the body the load of toxic substances in order to enhance treatment results. The belief is that detoxification is a decisive step towards restoration of the body's regulatory mechanism and reversal of diseased cells to the behaviour of normal cells, which are programmed to die when they have fulfilled their task. The cell death is called apoptosis. With all detoxification patients, whether they suffer from cancer or chronic degenerative diseases, the function of the liver, kidneys, colon, lungs, skin, and lymph system is informed by herbal preparations, supplementation of nutrients, high fluid intake, lymph drainage for infrared sauna, etc., according to individual needs. The liver fulfills many vital functions—digestive, hormonal, and others—and it is responsible for the proper functioning of the organisms in general. It represents the body's major detoxification system. The liver removes toxic substances that have been ingested, such as food additives, harmful minerals, toxic medication, etc. It extracts from the blood the residues and waste material resulting from cellular breakdown and transforms them into byproducts that can be excreted by the intestine or kidneys to aid in healing.

Beta-sitosterol: One of the very best studies done was published in the *British Journal of Urology*, volume 80 (1997), at the University of Dresden. Drs. Klippel, Hilti, and Schipp studied 177 men for six months who suffered from BPH. Half the men got the prescription extract Azuprostat containing 130 mg of beta-sitosterol. They cited a full thirty-two references to substantiate their research. They concluded by suggesting, "These results show that beta-sitosterol is an effective option in treatment of BPH." Beta- sitosterol supplement has also been used by both men and women to promote healthy cholesterol and triglyceride levels. A research article suggested that years ago studies showed its effect with no change in diet or exercise. Over fifty articles have been published in international medical journals for studies done on both humans and laboratory animals. Beta-sitosterol may be difficult to find in drug stores or health food stores. The oil, a constituent of a few plants, including soy beans and pygeum, contains a mixture of phytosterols, a hormone called beta-sitosterol. Studies validate a minimum of twenty mg per day of beta-sitosterol to increase urine flow and decrease residual urine volume significantly, research suggests that beta-sitosterol inhibits prostaglandin synthesis, thus reducing inflammation.

Flax seed oil: Flax seed oil, which contains omega-3 fatty acids, is recommended as very good for prostate health. There are several articles with information on the healing properties of flax seed oil. The essential fatty acids in flax seed oil are the key healing components. Essential fatty acids (EFAs) are needed by the body; the body cannot function efficiently without them. Essential fatty acids work throughout the body to protect cell membranes, providing healthy substances while keeping out unhealthy substances. Flax seed oil is a blue plant, and its natural oil (also known as linseed oil) is highly recommended for its therapeutic and nutritious benefit on the whole body.

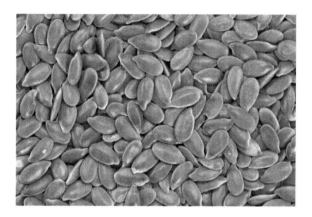

Nettle: Nettle is suggested to be an energy stimulant and can be used as support for joints. It is a diuretic astringent herb with tonic properties, used to reduce blood pressure. The roots have similar properties and are used to reduce prostate enlargement. Nettle leaves also have properties of minerals, flavonol glycosides, phenolic acid amines, beta-sitosterol and tannins.

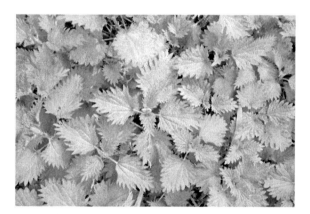

Pygeum Bark: The bark of this tree is said to contain lipophilic sterols, including beta- sitosterol and sitosterol plus unique fatty acids. These ingredients influence prostaglandin synthesis to help control the damaging effects of inflammation. Studies suggest that pygeum decreases androgen levels, resulting in less prostate exposure to hormones. Other components of pygeum help prevent swelling of soft tissue. Chemical analysis and pharmacological studies conclude that lipophilic extract of pygeum bark has three categories of active constituents. The phytosterols, including beta-sitosterol, have anti-inflammatory effects by interfering with the formation of pro-inflammatory effects. They interfere with the formation of pro-inflammation prostaglandins that tend to accumulate in the prostates of men with benign prostatic hyperplasia (BPH). The pentacyclic terpenes have an anti-edema or decongesting effect. The last group is the ferulic esters. These constituents are said to reduce levels of the hormone prolactin and also block cholesterol in prostate. Prolactin increases uptake of testosterone in the prostate, and cholesterol increases uptake of testosterone and its more active form of dihydrotestosterone.

Soy isoflavones: Soy isoflavones has shown great value for treatment of the prostate. There are numerous studies suggesting that soy isoflavones have value to prostate health. The main constituents in soy are genistein and daidzein. Studies on prostate health and soy isoflavones have been published in journals such as *Prostate, Anticancer Research, Journal of Endocrinology, Nutrition and Cancer, Journal of Steroid Biochemistry,* and other journals. The research has shown that genistein, a prominent phytoestrogen component of soybeans, has been identified with multifunction related to cancer prevention. Scientific investigation suggests that genistein can slow down the rate of cell division, block the growth of new blood vessels, ground the cancer cells (anti-angiogenesis), suppress the growth of human breast and prostate cancer, and inhibit the enzyme (5 alpha-reductase) that converts testosterone to dihydrotestosterone. All of these metabolic effects are associated with a reduced risk of prostate cancer growth and progression.

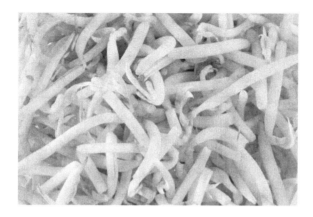

Garlic: The *American Journal of Clinical Nutrition* published a study in 1997 showing the value of garlic supplementation for prostate health. There are articles also suggesting that garlic is good for cardiovascular health. Garlic has antibiotic properties. Researchers also suggested that garlic and onions prevent men from developing prostate cancer. Benefits could be due to alliums, a sulphur-based compound that is responsible for the high smell. Recent studies have shown that foods high in lycopene, such as tomatoes, as well as the active sulfur compounds in garlic, onions, leeks, shallot, and chives may all be potentially beneficial treatment for prostate cancer.

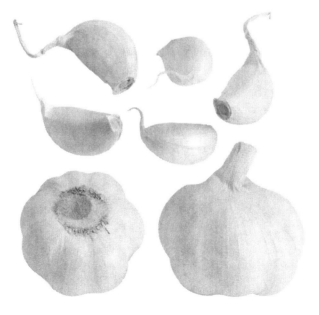

A study in the *Journal of the National Cancer Institute* showed that men who ate more than a third of an ounce (nine grams) a day from the allium food group were about 50 percent less likely to have prostate cancer than those who ate less of these foods.

Green Tea Extract: The healing properties of green tea extract for prostate health have been recorded by the *Journal of the National Cancer Institute* and *Cancer Letters*, which stated that the human body constantly produces unstable molecules called oxidants or free radicals. These free radicals damage cell proteins and genetic materials. This damage may leave the cells and tissues vulnerable to cancer. Green tea extract provides antioxidants that allow the human mind/body to scavenge and selectively inhibit specific enzymes activities that lead to cancer.

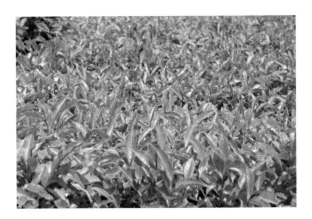

Citrus Pectin: Citrus pectin has been shown to have value in treating prostate cancer. Studies have been published in the *Journal of the National Cancer Institute* and *Biochemical Molecular Biology International* showing the anticancer properties of citrus pectin. The recommended dose is five grams per day in juice. Pectin is a soluble fiber that is found in most plants but is most concentrated in citrus fruits and apples. Pectin is obtained from the citrus peels of fruits and apple pulp. For therapy, pectin can be used in combination with the clay kaolin (hydrated aluminum silicate) for the management of diarrhea and elevated cholesterol.

Quercetin: It is suggested that some preliminary laboratory studies indicated that quercetin may inhibit the growth of prostate cancer cells in test tubes. However, at this time, it is relatively unknown how this will translate to prevention and treatment of prostate cancer. Quercetin, which is primarily found in apples, onions, and black tea, is a type of flavonoid (plant pigment) that serves as a building block for other members of the flavonoid family. Quercetin has been suggested to help fight a host of disorders, such as asthma, cancer, and heart disease. It is an antioxidant that combats the destructive free radical molecules that contribute to many degenerative diseases. Among people with high dietary intakes of quercetin and other major flavonoids, some studies show lower rates of prostate and other cancers such as lung, breast, and pancreatic cancer.

Glutathione: A Chinese study showed the importance of glutathione levels for prostate health in the journal *Shondong Yike Daxue Xuebo*. Glutathione levels are critical for immunity and how long you live. The study suggested too that glutathione is expensive; therefore taking about a 600-mg capsule of N-acetyl-cysteine will enhance your glutathione level effectively. You will gain many benefits by raising your glutathione levels, such as raising your immunity to fight disease. Selenium is an important constituent of the body's naturally produced antioxidant glutathione peroxidase, and its cancer-preventative effect may be associated with increased glutathione levels.

Lobelia: Lobelia helps lessen one's desire for nicotine/smoking addiction, reduces cravings and nervousness, bronchitis, asthma, meningitis, hepatitis, muscle problems, is the most powerful relaxant among herbs, prevents lockjaw, helps adrenal glands, is a tonic for kidneys, prostate glands, the reproductive, circulatory, and nervous systems, and grows a very deep top root (estimated at between twenty and seventy feet deep), thus gaining access to minerals and nutrients that may not be found in depleted topsoil.

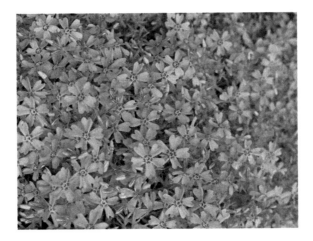

Cascara Sagrada: Cascara sagrada must be "whole leaf" and is used for abdominal pain, colitis, appendicitis, Crohn's Disease, or inflammatory/irritable bowel. It is suggested that it is an excellent laxative and a good colon cleanser and is used for parasites, cancer, liver disease, constipation (taken in the evening for elimination in the morning), and a tonic for the liver, gall bladder, and digestive system. To be effective during illness, take over 3,000 mg/day of the clear gel layer for three to six months, and for maintenance 1,000 mg/day. It is suggested that since the potency is difficult to get affordably in supplement form and the taste can be difficult to swallow, you can also take eight oz/day of whole-leaf aloe vera gel that has bitter constituents removed.

Alfalfa: Alfalfa is one of the most nutritious foods known. It possesses anti-aging properties and is used to effectively treat arthritis, anemia, rheumatism, and cancer, as a blood purifier, for morning sickness, high cholesterol, and high blood sugar, as a liver detoxifier, antibiotic, laxative, antitumor properties, and for chlorophyll. It contains more protein and calcium than beef, milk, and eggs, contains every essential amino acid, and is useful for kidney stones, diabetes, treating hyperactive/overactive thyroid-stimulating hormones, strengthening heartbeat, and reducing the rate of heartbeat.

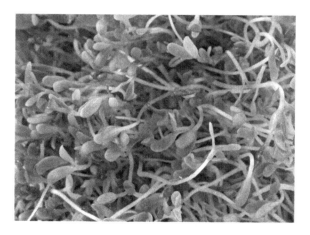

Burdock Root: Burdock root is suggested as one of the best blood purifiers, effective in all skin disease, syphilis, rheumatism, indigestion, kidney disease, scrofula, canker sores, scurvy, gonorrhea, eczema, leprosy, boils, measles, vertigo, hives, dandruff, sore throat, insect bites, snake bites, and dropsy. It has anti-bacterial, anti-fungal, and anti-cancer properties, contains polyacetylenes, amino acids, and insulin, and restores harmony to the body. It stimulates bile and acts as a liver cleanser and as a blood purifier. It promotes kidney function and helps filter blood.

Parsley: Parsley stimulates the menstrual cycle, is good for flatulence and colic, and is a breath freshener. It is very rich in iron, potassium, vitamin C, and vitamin A and is excellent for dropsy, jaundice, gallbladder stones, cancer, and venereal diseases. A poultice of the bruised leaves is excellent when applied to swollen prostate glands and other glands. Do not dilute the gel by taking it with juice or drinking shortly before or after ingesting the gel. Each ounce is usually equivalent to about 400. Parsley is historically famous and was used by such ancient herbalists as Hippocrates, Dioscorides, and Gerard. As a member of the carrot family, it was valued as a culinary spice and medicine.

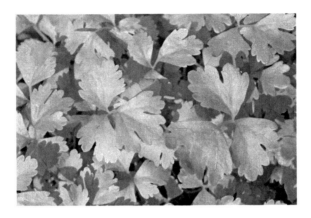

Juniper Berries: The juniper berry is one of the herbs that is recommended for prostate therapy. Juniper berries are suggested to be helpful in support of high blood pressure, congestive heart failure, arthritis, nerve pain, rheumatism, gout, and cystitis. A valuable item of commerce, the oil of juniper berries is a prime ingredient in the alcoholic beverage gin. The ripe berries have been used for their antiseptic properties in various kinds of urinary infections, as a diuretic, and in conditions such as prostatitis

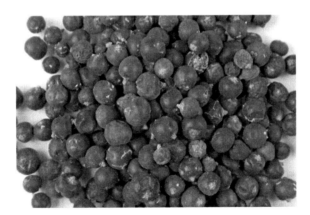

Pumpkin Seeds (Curcurbita Pepo): A good source of zinc and essential fatty acids, nutrients which promote prostate health, they also contain curcurbitin and phytosterin. It is recorded that in the early 1900s, pumpkin seeds were used to treat enlarged prostate symptoms and other urinary tract complications. Pumpkin seeds are suggested to contain protective phytosterol compounds, which may be responsible for shrinking the prostate. Pumpkin seeds and the oil they contain have long been used as a nutrient and medicine. They have been the subject of a number of studies to identify their health-promoting properties. Preliminary studies have shown that pumpkin may help to reduce hormonal damage to prostate cells and could prevent the risk of developing prostate cancer.

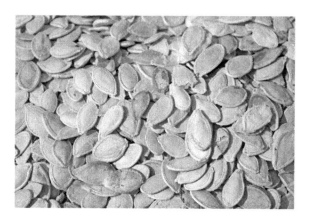

Cellular Zeolite: Cellular zeolite is promoted as an excellent cancer-fighting product. It is excellent for detoxification and also improves the alkalinity of your mind/body. Cellular zeolite works by allowing the zeolite to travel throughout the mind/body and get into the cells. Zeolite is a negative-charged mineral that naturally attracts toxins, which are positively charged, to it and traps them in its cagelike structure. Zeolite molecules normally become quite large because they stack together very easily. Studies show that when you take measured quantity of cellular zeolite, 40 percent shows up in the stools and 60 percent in the urine, which suggest that it gets into the bloodstream and goes throughout the body.

Lipid (1992), JNIC vol. 27, pp. 798-803, shows that fat intake as well as obesity were major causes of prostate disease and backs this up with fifty-nine references. Omega-3 fatty acids inhibited cancer while omega-6 stimulated it. This is further proof that vegetable oils could be detrimental for you as they mainly are made up of omega-6 fatty acids.

Fish Oils: Does fish oil cause or prevent prostate cancer? Report shows that a prestigious team of researchers from the National Cancer Institute, the Harvard Medical School, the Harvard School of Public Health, and Karolinska Institute in Stockholm released a report on the study of ALA, fish oil, and other fatty acids and their effect on prostate health. Alpha-linolenic acid (ALA) is a major component of flax seed oil. Some studies have shown that a high intake of ALA is associated with an increased risk of prostate cancer. The study involved 47,866 male American health professionals who were studied over a fourteen-year period beginning in 1986. They completed detailed food frequency questionnaires from 1996 to 2000. Within those fourteen years, 2,965 new cases of prostate cancer had been reported, with 448 of these being advanced (metastasized) or fatal. The total incidence of prostate cancer developed over the fourteen-year period was 0.5 percent per year.

"The researchers found no correlation between ALA intake and overall prostate cancer risk, but did observe a strong association between a high ALA intake and the risk of advanced prostate cancer. Men with a high ALA intake (greater than 0.58 percent of energy or about 1.3 grams/day) were twice as likely to develop advanced prostate cancer as were men with a lower intake (less than 0.37 percent of energy or about 0.8 grams/day) after adjusting for all other known variables that could affect the risk. The risk was slightly higher for ALA from non-animal sources than for ALA from meat and dairy sources. There was a trend for red meat, mayonnaise, and salad dressings to be associated with a high risk. The intake of two other abundant fatty acids, linoleic acid and arachidonic acid, was not related to prostate cancer risk."

The same team of researchers suggested that they found a protective effect associated with a high intake of fish oils—eicosapentaenoic acid (EPA) and docosahexaenoic acid (DHA). They suggested that men with a daily intake of 470 mg/day were 11 percent less likely to develop prostate cancer than were men with an intake of less than 125 mg/day. The beneficial effect of EPA plus DHA was particularly pronounced in regard to the incident of advanced prostate cancer. The report stated that fish oil supplements were slightly less effective than fish oil from fatty fish. The report may be indicating that vitamin D and vitamin A are needed to obtain the maximum benefit.

Fighting Cancer by Increasing Cellular Oxygen: There is a research theory that suggested that one of the underlying causes of cancers may be low cellular oxygenation levels. The low oxygenation level in new cells damages their cellular respiration enzymes, and this could cause them to become cancerous. The respiratory enzymes in the cells, which make energy aerobically using oxygen, die when cellular oxygen levels drop. When this happens the cells can no longer produce energy aerobically; therefore if the cells are to live, they must partially ferment sugars, producing energy anaerobically. To maintain optimum health, every cell in our body must have a continuous supply of oxygen. When the oxygen is in short supply, changes begin to take place in the cells. They do not perform efficiently and their functions are ineffective. All physical and chemical processes within our body require oxygen. It is imperative to maintain a balanced internal environment to keep our blood purified. Short supply of oxygen will allow carbon dioxide to build up within our system. It is important to understand that our body uses oxygen and nutrients within the bloodstream to nourish the whole mind-body, and more oxygen is needed to rid itself of toxic waste products that contribute to diseases. If carbon dioxide is allowed to build up within our system, its toxic nature causes cells to degenerate, and lead to weakening of the immune system. With my engineering background, it is easy for me to understand the danger of build-up of dissolved oxygen in our system. Build-up of dissolved oxygen in a steam generator will corrode boiler tubes and other metals. When the tubes and metals are corroded, they will over-heat, rupture and explode. Therefore, an efficient oxygen scavenging system has to be installed to eliminate dissolved oxygen. Oxygen is imperative for life. However, its residue must be eliminated from our system in an efficient manner to prevent damage to our internal environment. Oxygen and nutrients provide energy for the cells, although there may not be perfect efficiency in their delivery to all cell, tissues and relevant parts. There must be energy balance to prevent biochemical accidents in the physical and chemical development of our metabolic process.

Dr Warburg, winner of the 1931 Nobel Prize for proving that cancer is caused by lack of oxygen respiration in cells, stated in one of his articles that "the cause of cancer is no longer a mystery. We know it occurs whenever any cell is denied 60% of its oxygen. Cancer, above all other diseases, has countless secondary causes. But, even for cancer, there is only one primary cause. Summarized in a few words, the primary cause of cancer is the replacement of the respiration of oxygen in normal body cells by a fermentation of sugar. All normal body cells meet their energy needs by respiration of oxygen, whereas cancer cells meet their energy needs in great part by fermentation. All normal cells are thus obligate aerobes, whereas all cancer cells are partial anaerobes."

It is suggested by researchers that some causes of poor oxygenation include a buildup of carcinogens and other toxins within and around cells, which block and then damage the cellular oxygen-respiration mechanism. Clumping up of red blood cells slows down the bloodstream and restricts flow to capillaries. The restriction is also the cause of poor oxygenation. Whenever there is restriction in our circulatory system, there is a problem. That's because diseases start at the cellular level. The body needs energy to function at optimum efficiency, and oxygen is one of the most important requirements for life. This is why many of our health care practitioners place so much emphasis on the amount of oxygen we are receiving. The deficiency of clean air in our communities can be attributed to many of our illnesses. Also, processed foods, added chemicals to preserve these foods, refined corroborates, saturated fats, alcohol, excessive caffeine, soda pop, cigarettes, and similar unhealthy products in our consumer society are a detriment to our well being. All these, combined with environmental pollution, and toxic chemicals used both at home and in the workplace result in great stress on our digestive and metabolic systems.

The nutritional biochemistry and metabolic pathway of the body's natural state, particularly where nutrient availability is altered, provide room for disease. The function of the metabolic pathway is to break down complex substances to more simple compounds, for example, protein to amino acids, the reverse process is the synthesis of simple compounds to a more complex molecular process.

The breakdown reactions are called catabolism and anabolism. Catabolism is the breakdown of complex compounds into simpler compounds. This includes the digestion of food into smaller molecules, and the release of energy from these molecules within the cells. Anabolism is the building of simple compounds into substances needed for cellular activities and growth and repair of tissues.

Another way of looking at the same reaction is the standard free energy changes that occur during their course of action, to drive them into energy-yielding or energy-using reactions.

Overall, as mentioned before, perfect efficiency may not be achieved. However, there should be energy-balanced within the cells. This is why a cell never carries out two types of reactions in isolation from each other. Energy-yielding ones are always linked to energy-using reactions and one is used to drive the other. In any one pathway the two types of reactions are found to be linked to a common chemical intermediate, which processes a highly reactive group. The intermediate, with its reactive group, is formed at the expense of a small number of compounds, ubiquitously present in the cell, (existing or being in all places at the same time). There are three types of such small groups of transfer molecules. The most important of all the group transfer molecules is adenosine triphosphate (ATP).

ATP is considered by biologists to be the energy currency of life. It is the energy molecule that stores the energy we need to do almost all activity for life. ATP is present in every cell, and essentially all the physical and chemical reactions that require energy for operation is obtained directly from stored ATP. As food in the cells are gradually oxidized, the released energy is used to restore the ATP so that the cells always maintain a supply of this essential molecule. When several sequences of molecules are linked together, they are referred to as macromolecules. The most significant thing about these giant molecules is that they posses a certain individuality that the simple substances lack. Two molecules of glucose or of ATP are identical to whatever source they are prepared from. Two molecules of copper, sulphate or water are broken down in a similar way. However, within the long chains of repeatedly linked units that comprise the macromolecules, there is room for a variety of mistakes or mutation. What's important is the precision and variation in the structure of molecules. One such case is that of hemoglobin, a blood protein that contains over three hundred amino acids. If the sequence is changed by having a single amino acid out of sequence, the hemoglobin won't function properly. This results in the previously mentioned disease known as sickle cell anemia. There are many similar cases of large chains of molecules substituting themselves in any sequence, that determine whether we live or die from diseases.

In our chemistry of life, surgery, physical therapy, drugs, osteopathy, massage, acupuncture, homeopathy, supplements, herbal support, and all other healing therapies have their rightful place. Yet, no healing remedy can be successful without adequate nutritional support for our mind-body. Only natural God-given foods build, strengthen and repair damaged tissues, and provide energy for operation and maintenance of the whole human body.

Getting oxygen into the cells is difficult, and most approaches do not work well. Breathing oxygen is limited by the amount of hemoglobin available and the acidity levels. According to Warburg, it is the increased amount of carcinogens, toxicity, and pollution that cause cells to be unable up take oxygen efficiently. Research shows that the majority of the food and drinks we consume are acidic. Many of us allow our body to become oases of toxic waste that could shut down many of our organs that provide house-cleaning duties. We must regularly eliminate unwanted toxic wastes that are corrosive to our cells, tissues and system. Disease of the human body starts at the cellular level. It's important to note that efficient performance of cells are very critical to optimal health. One of the areas of concern is the internal environment of alkalinity and acidity. Our internal environment should be more alkaline than acidic. Too much acid in the body provides an environment for cells to become cancerous. In engineering we have to maintain our boiler feed water pH at neutral or alkaline to prevent corrosion of boiler tubes and metals. In life we must consume food that will not allow our body to be too acidic. There is a biological set point in our body that provides equilibrium. If there is too much deviation from the set point, efficient operation of our whole body is at risk. If your car is out of balance it does not function at optimum efficiency. Our body is no different. Its physical and chemical concentration and reactance, acidity and alkalinity are critical to actions carried out. Deviation causes critical changes to occur in the behavior of this highly complex process. When oxidization is being carried out, all processes must follow proper sequence to provide an accident-free, biochemical operation.

According to Keiichi Morishita in his book, *Hidden Truth of Cancer*, as blood starts to become acidic, the body deposits acid substances in the cells to get them out of the blood. This allows the blood to remain slightly alkaline; it also causes the cells to become more acidic and toxic, which may result in a decrease in oxygen levels. To alleviate this problem you should eat more alkaline rich food to allow your body to be more alkaline.

Hormones Support: It is a known fact that hormones have some influence on the health of the prostate. This knowledge has generated much controversy and misleading information. It has been suggested by conventional practitioners that testosterone is the fuel that ignites the growth of the prostate and prostate cancer. However, the question arises why younger men with high testosterone levels are not likely to have benign prostate or prostate cancer and older men with low testosterone develop benign or prostate cancer. When testosterone levels become low in older men, their estrogen level rises and their DHEA is depleted. This would suggest that it is not the testosterone itself that causes the problem. It is most likely contributed to the low level of testosterone, their high estrogen level, and the reduction of other essential hormones. If testosterone were the cause of prostate cancer, young men would be dying from prostate cancer. Many studies have shown that men with the highest level of testosterone have the least prostate enlargement and men with the highest level of estrogen have enlarged prostates.

Progesterone: The ability of progesterone to prevent and reverse prostate cancer has been highly reported by Dr. John Lee and many well-known physicians and natural health practitioners for many years.

It is difficult to understand why the medical establishment places the blame for prostate problems on testosterone and why they are not supportive of progesterone treatment. Natural progesterone should not be mistaken for synthetic progestins. They are molecularly different, and natural progesterone does not carry the same side effects or risks that the synthetic one does.

Men produce estrogen (Estradiol), but in lower amounts than women. Many scientists and researchers have suggested the importance of the testosterone and estrogen ratio to normal prostate or diseased prostate. Men also produce progesterone, but only about half the amount produced by females. Progesterone is normally produced in men by the adrenal glands and testes. Unfortunately, male progesterone levels drop with aging, just as male testosterone does. It is suggested by scientists that severe, prolonged stress could also deplete progesterone. Progesterone is vital to good health in humans. It is suggested by scientists that it is the primary precursor of our adrenal cortical hormones and testosterone. The male hormone testosterone is antagonist to estradiol. Testosterone prevents estradiol from causing prostate cancer by destroying the prostate cancer cells it stimulates. Research studies have also shown that when prostate cells are exposed to estrogen, the cells proliferate and become cancerous. When progesterone or testosterone was added, cancer cells died.

DHEA (Dehydroeplandrosterone): DHEA is the most abundant steroid in the body, and it declines with age. Abnormally low levels have been reported to be related to a number of degenerative diseases, including cancer. Supplemental DHEA has been cited in several reports to have anticancer activity. DHEA, melatonin, and pregenolone levels fall very low in men after age forty. LH (luteinizing hormone) and FSH (follicle-stimulating hormone) rise in men as they age, which could cause problems in men's health. It is recommended that if your DHEA is low you should supplement it with twenty-five mg of DHEA, and you should monitor your level every three to six months.

Researchers suggest that there is increasing evidence that nutrition may play a significant role in the prevention and/or progression of prostate cancer. There are data to suggest that diet may be of more significance in the behaviour of prostate cancer than in either breast or colon cancer. Autopsy studies have demonstrated that there is evidence of microscopic prostate cancer cells in approximately 80 percent of men over eighty years old. This finding is the same throughout the world and is unrelated to race. However, the incidence of clinically significant prostate cancer is significantly greater in Western countries as opposed to Oriental countries. In a study published in the *British Journal of Cancer* in 1991 by Dr. Schimizu and Associates, it was noted that within one generation, there was a fourfold to ninefold increase in prostate cancer among men who immigrated to the United States in contrast with their counterparts who remained in Japan. In a similar study published in *Acta Oncologica* in 1991 by Dr. Muir and Associates, there was found a threefold to sevenfold increase in the incidence of prostate cancer in Oriental men who immigrated to the San Francisco Bay area. This suggests the presence of either an environmental or nutritional factor that may be playing a role in stimulating the growth of microscopic cancer cells to clinically significant cancer in the United States, Canada, and some European countries.

Abstract from the Journal of Nutrition suggested that; "Because of their safety and the fact that they are not perceived as "medicine," food-derived products are highly interesting for development as chemopreventive agents that may find widespread, long-term use in populations at normal risk. Numerous diet-derived agents are included among the 40 promising agents and agent combinations that are being evaluated clinically as chemopreventive agents for major cancer targets. These targets include breast, prostate, colon and lung. Examples include green and black tea polyphenols, soy isoflavones, Bowman-Birk soy protease inhibitor, curcumin, phenethyl isothiocyanate, sulforaphane, lycopene, indole-3-carbinol, perillyl alcohol, vitamin D, vitamin E, selenium and calcium. Many food-derived agents are extracts, containing multiple compounds or classes of compounds. For developing such agents, the National Cancer Institute (NCI) has advocated codevelopment of a single or a few putative active compounds that are contained in the food-derived agent. The active compounds provide mechanistic and pharmacologic data that may be used to characterize the chemopreventive potential of the extract, and these compounds may find use as chemopreventives in higher risk subjects (patients with precancers or previous cancers). Other critical aspects to developing the food-derived products are careful analysis and definition of the extract to ensure reproducibility (e.g., growth conditions, chromatographic characteristics or composition), and basic science studies to confirm epidemiologic findings associating the food product with cancer prevention."

Of all these potential factors related to prostate cancer, the most significant has been the relationship between dietary fat and prostate cancer. Among animal fat, fat from red meat was most strongly linked to advanced cancer. Those who consumed the most red meat were said to be two-and-a-half times more likely to have advanced cancer or to die from prostate cancer, than those who ate meat infrequently. The investigators of this report found a tenfold difference intake of animal fat between low and high consumers, ranging from an average of 3.2 grams of fat from red meat each day to 30.5 grams per day. Fat intake was also associated with the risk of advanced cancer. Those who consumed an average of 88.6 grams of fat per day had a 76 percent greater chance of developing advanced prostate cancer, than those who averaged 53.2 grams of fat daily. There have been several well-executed studies involving more than 3,000 patients with prostate cancer and more than 4,600 patients without prostate cancer. Eleven of these studies have shown a positive association between increased dietary fat and a higher risk of prostate cancer, with some studies showing a greater than threefold increase in cancer incidence. In another group of studies of close to 100,000 men, there was also a positive association between dietary fat and the development of prostate cancer. In a recent study published in the *Journal of the National Cancer Institute* in 1993 by Dr. Giovannucci and Associates, there was a marked increase in the likelihood of prostate cancer in men with a high dietary fat intake from red meat. These investigators found a strong relationship between the intake of linolenic acid, a fatty acid primarily associated with red meats, and prostate cancer. But Dr Giovannucci said most of this fatty acid was derived from animal fats rather than vegetable oils in men's diets. He also suggested that there is a need for more research. When assessing this information, we must take into account, the fact that there are good fats and there are bad fats. There are essential fats the human body needs for survival…

There is a considerable amount of research available proving the existence of links between specific types of food and cancer. These links exist both for cancer in general and for prostatic cancer in particular. Way back in 1982, the National Research Council in the United States published a technical report entitled "Diet Nutrition and Cancer," which showed that diet was probably the single most important factor in the development of cancer and that there was evidence linking cancer of the breast, colon, and prostate to particular foods or types of food. But the evidence linking cancer and food goes back many years before 1982. For example, since the mid-1970s there has been strong evidence to show a link between a high fat intake and a high risk for prostate cancer. Studies in forty-one countries have shown a high correlation between mortality from prostate cancer and the intake of fats, milk, and meats (especially beef). In 1993 a study of 47,855 men reported in a medical research modernization committee report revealed that men who ate a high-fat diet had a relative risk of 1-79 for advanced prostate cancer as compared to those on a low-fat diet. Men eating a high-fat diet are almost twice as likely to develop prostate cancer as men on the low fat-diet are. Dr Ernst Wynder, director of the American Health Foundation called for more aggressive intervention studies in which men with early prostate cancer would be placed on a carefully controlled low-fat diet to see if it reduced their chance of dying of prostate cancer. Such a study was about to be done by the foundation, scrutinizing 2,000 women who had been treated for early-stage breast cancer. I have not seen the findings from this study.

Numerous studies have shown that a high intake of tomatoes markedly reduces the risk of prostate cancer. It is believed that this beneficial effect is due to lycopene, the most common carotenoid in tomatoes. A team of researchers from Wayne State University, McGill University, the University of Maryland, has concluded a clinical trial aimed at evaluating the benefits of lycopene supplementation in prostate cancer patients. The study included twenty-six men with clinical localized prostate cancer who were scheduled to undergo radical prostatectomy. The men randomized into a control group and an intervention group. The intervention group received one fifteen mg lycopene capsule with breakfast and dinner for three weeks prior to surgery. Blood samples were taken before the start of the supplementation and three weeks prior to surgery. They removed the tumor, and surrounding tissue was examined by pathologists. The researchers conclude that lycopene supplementation lowers PSA levels. They observed an average of an 18 percent decrease in the lycopene group as compared to a 14 percent increase in the control group. The level of the tumor-suppressing protein CX43 in the malignant part of the tumor was found to be substantially higher in the lycopene group. It was also apparent that tumors tended to be smaller and more sharply defined (less encroachment into surrounding healthy tissue) in the lycopene group. No adverse effects of lycopene supplementation were reported by the patients or the physicians. The researchers conclude that lycopene is likely to be beneficial for both prevention and treatment of prostate cancer, but they urge larger trials to confirm this.

In Staffordshire, in the UK, British researchers have confirmed that exposure to sunlight helps prevent prostate cancer. Their study involved 210 men diagnosed with prostate cancer and 155 men with an enlarged prostate, but no prostate cancer (controls). The men were interviewed in order to estimate their lifetime sun exposure. Men with the lowest exposure were found to have a three-times greater incidence of prostate cancer than did men with high lifetime exposure. Sunburns in childhood were found to be particularly protective, with men having had one or more childhood sunburns being six times less likely to develop prostate cancer than did men who did not experience childhood sunburns. The researchers are not sure why sun exposure is protective, but speculate that vitamin D and the parathyroid hormone may somehow be involved.

Paracelsus a Swiss physician known as the Father of Pharmacology stated that "All that mankind needs for good health and healing is provided in nature – the challenge to science is find it." The answer to our health problem can be found in nature. They are our fruits, vegetables and herbs. Such as apples, pears, oranges, mangos, peaches and others. They bud from heads of green cabbages, cauliflower and is found in vine-ripened tomatoes and golden cantaloupes and many other green leafy vegetables.

There are studies that show that a shortage of metabolic enzymes can jeopardize our health. If we digest more enzymes from our foods, more metabolic enzymes are freed, to prevent disease and maintain health. Unfortunately, all processed food has been heated by one or more means, and thus all natural enzymes have been destroyed. Eating of more raw foods is the safest way to preserve the metabolic enzymes our mind-body needs for optimum health and wellness. Squandering our enzyme-making capability depletes our body's capacity to create and preserve the thousands of other enzymes in the systems of our body. As a consequence, enzymes activity throughout the entire mind-body, declines rapidly and the aging process accelerates at a much faster rate, thereby allowing room for disease. Research has shown that sprouted seeds have lots of enzymes. Sprouted seeds are also a great source of Vitamin C, Carotenoid A; and B Vitamins and Minerals. When foods are processed, about 30% to 85% of required nutrients are destroyed. The human body is designed to ingest living foods created by nature. Processed and chemically preserved foods are foreign to the body. These substances are toxic and stressful to the body's metabolic process. The body is forced to cope with them. Under these circumstances, it dos the best it can. Raw foods provide more energy and allow all the organs and systems of the mind-body to perform with optimum efficiency.

As foods are increasingly put to the test in clinical trials, more and more doctors are beginning to view nutritional therapy as a possible treatment for prostate cancer. Dr. Ernst Wynder, the late founder of the American Health Foundation, pioneered the term nutritional therapy, which is using specific foods to treat an actual illness or prevent a latent one from becoming full blown. The prevention is to avoid foods or substances that might cause cancer; for example, high-fat foods. Protection is taking foods for substances such as lycopene or soy that may actively protect you against a potentially cancerous process in your body.

According to the National Cancer Institute, about one-third of all cancer deaths are related to malnutrition. For cancer patients, optimal nutrition is important. Cancer can deplete our body's nutrients and cause weight loss. Cancer and cancer treatment can also have a negative effect on your appetite and on your body's ability to digest foods. This occurs when there is need for high nutrients and the body can only support low-nutrient intake. This leaves your body's defense system vulnerable and defenseless against pathogens, which attack our bodies daily and subject sensitive organs to diseases.

Scientific evidence suggest that about one-third of the cancer deaths that occur in the United States each year are due to nutrition and physical activity factors, including obesity, cigarette smoking, and behavioral factors. Certain dietary patterns can substantially affect our risk of developing cancer. To modify the risk for cancer, the introduction of a healthy diet and regular physical activity, starting from childhood and continuing through old age, is a recommendation for health promotion and treatment.

A ten-year Japanese study involving 122,261 men aged forty or older showed the inverse association between the daily intake of green and yellow vegetables and mortality from prostate cancer. In other words the more green and yellow vegetables you eat, the less likely you are to develop prostate cancer. Another study showed that vegetarian men were less likely to develop prostate cancer.

In a paper entitled "A Case Control Study of Prostate Cancer with Reference to Dietary Habits," which was published in the journal incidence of prostatic cancer in Japan had been about 0.4 per 100,000 male members of the population, but by 1963 it had increased to 2.0 per 100,000 and by 1975 to 2.5 per 100,000. Observers had suggested that this increase might be linked to the Westernization of Japanese eating habits. During recent years the consumption of fat, animal protein, eggs, dairy products, and oil has increased considerably in Japan.

And so these authors studied sufferers from prostatic cancer and patient suffering from benign prostatic hypertrophy in order to identify the risk factors for prostatic cancer. These researchers found that a low daily intake of beta-carotene was significantly correlated with prostatic cancer development. Carrots and other orange and yellow-orange fruits and vegetables and dark green leafy vegetables are excellent sources of beta-carotene.

A study known as the Selenium and Vitamin E Cancer Prevention Trial (SELECT) was launched Tuesday, July 24, 2001, by the National Cancer Institute and a network of research sites known as the Southwest Oncology Group (SWOG). The study is to determine whether selenium and vitamin E supplements can individually or together protect men against prostate cancer. This study takes in a lot of countries, including Canada, and is to continue for twelve years. It is suggested that selenium and vitamin E, both naturally occurring nutrients, are antioxidants. They are capable of neutralizing toxins known as "free radicals," which might otherwise damage the general material of the cells and possibly lead to cancer. SELECT followed up leads from two other prevention trials to test these nutrients as potential agents in other cancers. In the first, reported in 1996, selenium was tested in 1,000 men and women and was found ineffective at preventing a type of non-melanoma skin cancer. However, in the men who took the nutrient, the incidence of prostate cancer was decreased by 60 percent. In the second, reported in 1998, beta-carotene and vitamin E were tested in 29,000 Finnish men who smoked to see if it could prevent lung cancer. It did not; in fact, the smokers who took beta-carotene were more apt to develop lung cancer and die than were those who did not. But again reduction in prostate was observed—a 32 percent reduction among those who took vitamin E.

Those asked to participate in SELECT are men age fifty-five or older (age fifty or older for black men because black men have the highest incidence of prostate cancer in the world) who have never had prostate cancer, have had no other cancer except non-melanoma skin cancer, and are generally in good health. Participants will be assigned by chance to one of four groups. One will take 200 micrograms of selenium daily plus an inactive capsule or placebo that looks like vitamin E; another will take 400 milligrams of vitamin E daily along with a placebo that looks like selenium; another will get two placebos.

Men who join SELECT will not need to change their diet in any way, but they must stop taking any supplements they buy themselves that contain selenium or vitamin E. If the participants wish to take a multivitamin, SWOG will provide, without charge, a specifically formulated one that does not contain selenium or vitamin E. "SELECT is the critical next step for pursuing the promising lead we saw for the prevention of prostate cancer," said Dr. Leslie Ford, Associate Director for Clinical Research in NCI's division of cancer prevention. He states that the only way to determine the real value of these supplements for prostate cancer is to do a large clinical trial focused specifically on this disease. I am encouraged to see more doctors and researchers focusing on nutritional supplement for the prevention of prostate cancer and other diseases. However, there are many negatives that will bring about the wrong result of this trial and cause more damage than good to nutritional supplements, orthomolecular medicine, and nutrition.

The first negative is that the men will not have a change in diet—(SAD) standard American diet is the cause of many diseases. Dietary choices are linked to 70 percent of all diseases affecting Americans. "Let your food be your medicine and your medicine be your food." This quote from Hippocrates holds as true today as it did when he said it. However, with the industrialization of the new world these concepts have lost their meaning. The consequence has been the physical, mental, and spiritual aspects of our health. Most people don't even recognize the rapid deterioration that is taking place. While the industrial revolution has created a more convenient place to live, it has by the same token taken away the essential elements of life, the essential nutrients our bodies need to function properly.

No other generation before ours has been exposed to so many man-made chemicals and toxic substances. The air we breathe is polluted, the water we drink is not clean, the food we eat is processed, our lifestyle is sedentary, our body cells lack oxygen, vitamins, minerals, and enzymes, our organs of detoxification and excretion are overwhelmed, and our bodies are overloaded with waste products and toxic metabolites that render them vulnerable to all sorts of bacteria and viruses.

The human body possesses self-regulatory mechanisms that are self-healing as designed by God. A healthy body is capable of eliminating toxic substances generated by its normal function and imposed on it by an unnatural lifestyle. If the production of toxic metabolites and ingestion of toxic substances overwhelms the organs of detoxification and excretion, the body stores these substances in the connective tissues, which become impeded in their important tasks of regulation and defense. Imbalance results and malaise signals us that the body is trying to get rid of toxins and needs help. Our first aid to the body is to release it from the burden of waste and toxic substances so that its regulatory self-healing mechanism can function again.

Detoxification is a decisive step toward the restoration of the body's regulatory mechanism and the reversal of diseased cells to the behaviour of normal cells. Detoxification occurs on many other levels as well as physical; this process can help clear congestions, illnesses, and potential diseases. It can improve energy and rejuvenate and prevent degeneration. Detoxification allows people to give up old toxic habits such as tobacco, alcohol, junk food, and coffee. Giving up such unhealthy habits can be very difficult unless the body is first purified. Once the body is cleansed, the majority of people find these poisons, which they once craved, to be obnoxious. They find themselves desiring the healthy things of nature such as raw juicy fruits, crisp flavorful vegetables, raw nuts, and pure water. Detoxification permits years of accumulated metabolic wastes in the cells to begin to be eliminated and allows the gastrointestinal, immune, and other body systems a chance to rest and repair. Good nutrition, good health, and cancer prevention cannot be achieved simply by using two nutritional supplements to neutralize free radicals. Our bodies must be able to digest, absorb, and assimilate the nutrients at the cellular level and to efficiently dispose of the waste products produced in the metabolic processes.

When wastes have accumulated faster than the body can rid itself of them, the cells can no longer utilize nutrients efficiently, and they become compromised in their ability to stay healthy. This is evidenced by such symptoms as fatigue, indigestion, sluggish bowels, diarrhea, headaches, menstrual problems, depression, skin disorders, musculoskeletal aches and pains, and eventually degenerative diseases such as cancer, heart disease, diabetes, arthritis, colitis, allergies etc. After detoxification is accomplished the cells work much more efficiently and are better able to utilize the nutrients ingested. Many people experience dramatic improvements in the way they feel after just a few days of a detoxification program.

The second negative of SELECT is that each of us is unique and different from everyone else. You have your own likes and dislikes. Each of us has different fingerprints, voice, and outward appearance. We have our own special talents and abilities. Our body's appearance, though in many ways similar, is also quite different from every other person's in the same way that our body's nutritional needs are quite different from the next person's needs. Biochemically, you are an individual. Research suggests that some people may need from four to forty times the amount of certain nutrients as others do.

Dr. Williams contributed to the evolution of the understanding of the molecular origin of disease with the development of the concept of biochemical individuality. He described anatomical and physiological variations among people and how they related in their individual responses to the environment. He was the first to gain recognition for the term "biochemical individuality" and how this is related to differing nutritional needs for optimal function based upon the fact that individuals developed in different environments in vitro. Although identical twins share the same genes, their differing nutritional and developmental environments can result in different expressions of genes as they grow older. Human bodies are diverse. Heredity definitely plays a part in longevity, but it is not the main factor and is usually not the deciding one. Whatever genetics one inherits may set a theoretical upper limit on what one's body is capable of; however, this limit may be rarely achieved in practice. Someone with weak constitution who takes care of his/her body may live a longer, healthier life than someone with a strong constitution who abuses his/her body. We have the choice either to live up to our body's genetic potential or to sabotage it. It is in your best interest to enhance your body's genetic potential.

Genetic factors are connected not only to the physical characteristics of individuals, but also to their biochemical milieu. The biochemical pathway of the body has significant genetic variability in terms of transcriptional potential and in terms of individual enzyme concentrations, of receptory ligand affinities, and of protein transporter efficiency. Diseases such as cancer and others are associated with specific biochemical abnormalities, which are either causal or aggravating factors of the illness. Orthomolecular medicine holds the view that it is possible that the provision of vitamins, amino acids, trace elements, proteins, or fatty acids in amounts sufficient to correct biochemical abnormalities will be therapeutic in preventing or treating such diseases.

The third negative aspect of SELECT is that there are many processes within the body that help us to remain healthy and resistant to disease. Attacking the body is a wide range of enemies such as bacteria, viruses, fungi, and poisons; in addition, the body is being damaged by free radicals. What are these free radicals? Basically they are molecules that have been deprived of oxygen atoms and are therefore hungry for oxygen. They find this oxygen in the fats embedded in the walls of normal cells. They therefore have to attack the cell walls to get the oxygen they require. This damages and even kills the cell. Free radicals are themselves the normal byproduct of the body's chemical reactions —particularly those processes involved in eliminating potentially toxic cellular waste materials. The more toxic waste materials there are the more free radicals are created.

Free radicals are being formed all the time, and their impact is controlled by the body in a number of ways. One way is by repairing the cell-wall damage. As we have seen, vitamins A, C, and E and CoQ10, lipoic acid, glutathione, and selenium are important for this process. They can intercept the free radicals before they do any harm. They are called antioxidants because they help the body to protect itself. They neutralize the free radicals before they reach the cells' walls. Vitamins and minerals work synergistically by protecting the cells from oxidization. There are other antioxidants not mentioned. Vitamins and minerals have other effects as well as being antioxidants. There are also co-enzymes, which are organic molecules that are required by certain enzymes to carry out catalysis. Every bodily process requires the actions of enzymes, so it is obvious that if the body is to function well it will need to have a steady source of vitamins and minerals.

Free radicals are both enemy and friend, as the saying goes, and wherever there is smoke there is fire. Similarly, wherever there is disease and destruction, there are free radicals. We could not exist without them. Similar to antioxidants, some free radicals at a low level are signaling molecules—that is, they are responsible for turning on and off genes. Some free radicals such as nitric oxide and superoxide are produced in very high amounts by our immune cells to "poison" viruses and bacteria. Some free radicals kill cancer cells, and in fact many cancer drugs are actually designed to increase the production of free radicals in the blood. Clearly we need free radicals for our survival. Yet in less than a split second, free radicals can turn on us, making us sick and aging us before our time.

For the study of selenium and vitamin E to work as a prevention of prostate cancer, all the above mentioned have to be considered. To have optimum health, the whole body has to be treated; one organ should not be singled out for protection from free radical damage. And symptomatology must be a factor. We all differ nutritionally. We need the same food factors—e.g., protein, fats, minerals, vitamins, fiber, sunlight, water, and rest —but we do not all need them in the same proportions from the same sources. Our ability to digest, absorb, and assimilate nutrients varies widely from person to person. The most important nutrient for each of us is the one we don't have enough of. It is highly probable that if one is not taking some nutritional supplement, critical nutrients are missing from his/her body. The concept of SELECT is interesting, but the approach is debatable.

Most scientific research on nutritional value has shown negative results, because some researchers' hypotheses are flawed. Some are of good intention; however, they are designed to operate with the same intensity as drugs. Drugs are designed to work to provide immediate results. Natural healing is a slow process that works to support the body's need for specific food.

Nutritional, clinical research regarding the association between specific disease and nutritional variables provides many report summaries from randomized double-blind control in humans from observational (epidemiological) studies to uncontrolled studies, animal studies, and blind studies. These clinical reports contribute a lot of new insights to the field of nutrition. Unfortunately, they also bring with them a lot of misunderstanding. That is because the methods of studying drugs are not well suited to the study of natural food factors.

Researchers want to know the effects of taking one particular drug at a time. They want to be sure that any results they observe are caused specifically by the drug and not by any extraneous factors. Therefore, they study each drug in isolation from all others. This approach works well for artificial substances that are not normally present in the body. For nutrients, however, it is not ideal; there is no practical way to isolate one nutrient and study only its effect on the human mind/body. We consume a smorgasbord of nutrients every day, all of which contribute to health in some way. It would be difficult to construct a study in which one group received no potassium. There would be imaginably difficult consequences. The best study we can do is to study the effects of adding additional amounts of specific nutrients to those already consumed on a daily basis. Nutrients do not work in isolation from each other. It is not realistic, therefore, to study them as if they did. Food factors interact with and support each other like links in a chain.

To study nutrients one at a time is to try to fit them into the medical mold. In medicine it is assumed that each disease has a unique set of symptoms. Forty people with the same condition may require forty different variations in nutritional therapy. Medicine treats the disease, and nutrition treats the person who has the disease. Drugs and nutrients work in entirely different ways, so the way of studying them should be different also. Drugs interfere with biochemical reactions; nutrient support them. Unless a drug is totally ineffective, it will produce some kind of side effect in just about everyone who uses it.

Supplementary food factors, however, produce a result only if the person tested had a deficiency or pre-existing need that was not being met through diet. To give a particular vitamin to a group of people will produce nonuniform results. Those who needed it will get some response; those who did not need it will not show any change. There are widespread biological variances in both human beings and animals. Each of us is biochemically unique. One person's body may require six time as much of a particular nutrient as someone else's body. There is no "standard" amount of any nutrient that will be of benefit to everyone who needs it. Therefore, the people who are using nutritional therapy for the treatment of cancer need to understand the principles of how food and lifestyle changes can provide healing.

Chapter 7:
Preventative Maintenance and Management of Mind/Body:

As an operational power engineer with fourteen years experience in operating and maintaining a power-generating plant, I will take the opportunity to use two features of a power plant to illustrate a preventative maintenance program of health and wellness for mind/body the nutritional way.

First, the safest and most efficient and economical way of operating a power-generating plant is to set up a well-planned and organized functional preventative-maintenance program in which all safety equipment, controls, motors, pressure vessels, piping, and other accessories are maintained according to specification standards and procedures, as instructed by the manufacturers' manuals. Second, to monitor the operation of the power plant to prevent costly downtime, the plant must be equipped with all the bells and whistles needed to relay quick and precise signals to the operators regarding the state of the equipment, controls, motors, etc., minute by minute, twenty-four hours per day. All the expensive bells and whistles mean nothing if the operators are not trained to interpret and assimilate the signals, or if the operators ignore the signals. The safety of the power plant would be compromised.

Our Creator has designed the human body/mind with an extraordinarily intricate and sophisticated network of internal bells and whistles (cells, tissues, organs, and systems), operating synergistically in a harmonious manner capable of miraculous and extraordinary sustaining, maintaining, and healing of the mind/body under the most stressful and strenuous circumstances, without us knowing what is happening. There are times, however, when the body will send us signals that something is wrong, and we should be trained to interpret and assimilate these signals.

We have an immune system equipped with a group of biochemical cells, tissues, and organs strategically located throughout the mind/body. Constantly challenged, these cells work together harmoniously with the aid of the central nervous system, endocrine system, and other systems to detect any foreign substance in the body and defend and eliminate what does not belong.

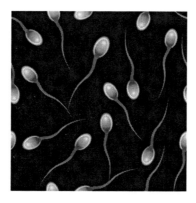

We are all formed from one single cell. The sperm from the father and the egg from the mother are united to form a single cell. Every cell in our body has forty-six chromosomes, except the sperm and the egg, which have twenty-three each. The sperm and the egg are joined together to form a cell, and immediately the cell starts to divide and multiply. It divides into two complete cells; these two cells become four, and the four become eight…etc. Soon the sperm divide and the egg multiplies to become an embryo with millions of cells, and the cells in the embryo divide and form into trillions of cells. The cells in the developing embryo are divided in an orderly way in a regulated and controlled process.

After the baby is born, the cells continue to rapidly multiply until the child reaches adulthood, and then normal growth is stopped. At this time the body will be made up of trillions of cells, which are the foundation and structure of the mind/body; however, cells will no longer multiply unless they are needed to replace damaged or worn-out cells or to repair tissues and organs.

How cells divide.

- One cell doubles by dividing into two
- Then four
- Then eight....

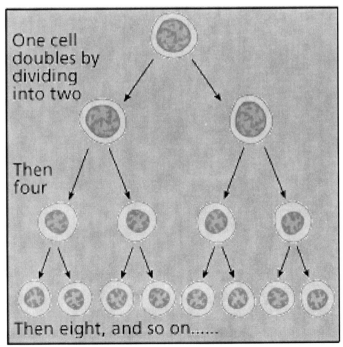

"Taken from CancerHelp UK"

Every normal cell contains twenty-three pairs of chromosomes. DNA is the controller and transmitter of genetic characteristics in the chromosomes we inherited from our parents and pass on to our children. DNA is the genetic blueprint of life.

Our chromosomes contain millions of cells and different messenger genes that tell the body how it should grow and function and behave. One gene tells our stomach how to make gastric juice; another tells the glands to secret the juice when food lands in the stomach.

Chromosome

- Cell nucleus
- Chromosome containing the genes

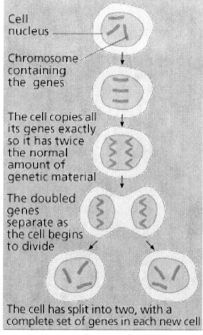

"Taken from CancerHelp UK"

Other genes determine the color of our eyes; another tells injured tissues how to repair themselves etc. Most of the time these genes function properly by sending the right messages. We remain in good health if everything is working as it should be. But there are an incredible number of genes and an unimaginable number of messages. Because the chromosomes reproduce themselves every time a cell divides, there are lots of opportunities for some things to go wrong.

At least a thousand times a day, clusters of bacteria, viruses, fungi, parasites, allergens, and other assorted organisms try to invade our body. We ingest bacteria; we pick up fungi; we inhale pollen. Not all these microorganisms are hostile. Some of these micro fibers live in us, and others live on us; others directly benefit us. Trillions of bacteria naturally occur in the intestine, and most help to protect our body from disease. They grow, reproduce, and feed on what we discard. Those that do pose a threat, however, are usually destroyed routinely, quietly, and unknown to us.

The immune system is naïve at first. It educates itself through each exposure to each new unknown invader. Without this system we could not survive. When the immune system malfunctions, we are vulnerable to a huge variety of disease from allergies to arthritis to cancer. Cancer results from genetic changes or damage to a chromosome within the cell.

Most of us carry within our bodies organisms that, if left unchallenged, would destroy us. They often live near us in a kind of stand-off relationship. They can overpower us if we are injured or weakened by stress, exhaustion, or malnutrition. Then the delicate balance is upset, and we become vulnerable to their attack and the many illnesses they unleash. When the human system functions normally, it can tell whether out-of-body invaders belong inside our body or not. When foreign invaders enter the bloodstream, they have surface-to-surface markers, which fit perfectly with certain immune system cells like a key fits a lock. This lets the immune system, in effect, fingerprint the invader cell, which in turn allows the immune system to distinguish self from nonself, which can be viral, bacterial, fungal, parasitic, chemical, or even a portion of the product of one of these organisms. The immune system can identify the precise nature of millions of intruders. Once it detects the intruders, it sets in motion a complex chain reaction designed to produce specific weapons to fight each of them. It is also designed to protect the body from further attack.

We all have different genetic materials that make up our immune systems; our cells must be cared for, nourished, and maintained in a proper biochemical environment. Our cells must be strengthened by essential factors such as natural food, clean water, sunlight, clean air, rest, meditation, relaxation, breathing, exercise, temperance, integrity, good mental, spiritual, and emotional attitudes, and a sense of purpose, a spiritual connection with God.

Our cells must be protected from today's environmental pollution, dietary stresses, toxic waste, toxic chemicals, toxic drugs, and stressful lifestyles, which frustrate and damage cellular function. These enemies of good health will make us more vulnerable, thereby allowing other undesirables to take over. This is why every person should have his/her individual preventative maintenance program, tailored to provide the mind and body with what it needs to function at optimum health and wellness.

To set up an effective functional preventative maintenance program we must have a nutritional plan and specification detailing every procedure, including safety against the standard American diet (SAD). Our body is equipped with early warning signals. These warning signals are complex. Therefore, special training is needed to detect the signals and determine the action to be taken, as mentioned before. Symptomatology and metabolic profiling are methods of reading these subtle signals and pinpointing potential problem areas. They involve answering approximately 600 questions about symptoms that may relate to nutrition imbalance. These questions are grouped together in relation to specific factors. A nutritional body appraisal is a useful tool in preventative healthcare and can help to design a personal program based on your unique biochemical individuality.

A good nutrition program begins with the understanding of how food affects the health and survival of the human mind and body. Symptomatology and metabolic profiling will determine the foods and supplements the human mind/body require to grow, reproduce, and maintain quality health. Listening to your body and providing it with all the essential factors will allow the body to maintain and cure itself of cancer and all degenerative diseases. Without food, our bodies could not stay warm or build or repair our cells, tissues, and organs or maintain a heartbeat. Eating the right food and supplements help us avoid certain diseases and recover faster from illness when it occurs. These and other important functions of our unique, intricate mind/body, organs, and systems of operation are fueled by chemical substances and nutrients, which provide harmonious healing by our well-tuned systems.

The nervous and endocrine systems work closely with the immune system, and their performances are critical to the functioning of the human mind and body, controlling growth, sexuality, learning, behaviour, reproduction, and much more. The nervous system is the controlling center of the mind/body. The endocrine system's main function is to produce and secrete hormones directly into the bloodstream that instruct cells what to do. The major organs of the endocrine system are the hypothalamus, the pituitary gland, the thyroid gland, the parathyroid gland and the islets of the pancreas, the adrenal glands, and the testes, which are affiliated with the prostate. The hormone system provides metabolism and cell function, controls the burning of fat, helps the body heal and rebuild, provides stamina and resistance to stress, and governs the reproductive system.

Brain cells

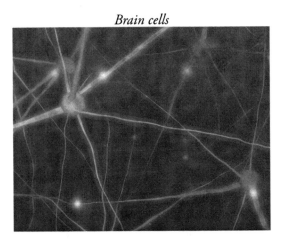

In the brain there are ten billion neurons (brain cells). Between each and every one of these are neurotransmitters. They are chemical messengers that transmit thoughts and mood from one cell to the next, allowing brains cells to communicate with each other. These neurotransmitters also send messages to the endocrine and immune systems and other systems. One of the fascinating things is that how we experience emotion and how we feel is dictated by certain neurotransmitters. Neurotransmitters change regularly between cells in your brain to meet the needs of your current circumstance. At night, to induce sleep, the brain needs to raise its level so certain thoughts are transmitted in a calming, quieting, and relaxing way for you to sleep well. In the morning it must lower its levels of these transmitters and raise excitatory transmitter levels. During exercise it increases levels of euphoria-inducing transmitters. During times of stress it must raise levels of another transmitter that helps you to remain alert and in control. When in pain, inhibitory transmitters are used by the brain to restrict the transmission of pain; the more present, the less pain you feel. It is critical that all of the major neurotransmitters be present daily and in sufficient amounts in order for the brain to be chemically balanced. When there are insufficient amounts of one or more of these it upsets the ratio and symptoms are experienced.

The endocrine system is a collection of glands that secrete chemical messages we call hormones. These signals are passed through the blood to arrive at target organs, which have cells processing the appropriate receptor. The role of the hormones is to select target cells and deliver the hormonal message on time and in precision. Hormones are grouped into three classes based on their structure:

1 steroid
2 peptides
3 amines

All three hormones work together harmoniously to provide a delicate balance. Steroids are lipids derived from cholesterol; peptides are short-chain amino acids. Most hormones are peptides. Amines are derived from the amino acid tyrosine and are secreted from the thyroid and adrenal medulla. The nervous system sends electrical messages to control and coordinate the mind/body; the endocrine system sends chemical messages and has receptors. The endocrine system's effects on the mind/body are wide reaching. Its message-sending ability influences the operations of all the body's tissues and organ systems.

For these systems and others to perform at optimum level they need nutrients. Nutrients are classified as proteins, essential fats, and carbohydrates, vitamins, minerals, fibers and water and include sunlight and clean air. When we eat a well-balanced meal, nutrients are released from foods through proper digestion. Digestion begins at the mouth by the action of chewing and the chemical activity of saliva—digestive fluids that contain enzymes, certain proteins that help break down food. Further digestion occurs as food travels through the stomach and small intestines where digestive enzymes and acids liquefy food and muscle contraction pushes it along the digestive tract. Nutrients are absorbed from the inside of the small intestine into the bloodstream and carried to every site in the body where they are needed. As these chemical reactions occur that ensure the growth and function of body tissues, the parts of the food that are not absorbed continue to move down the intestinal tract and are eliminated as feces.

Nutrients are classified as essential or nonessential. Nonessential nutrients are manufactured in the body and do not need to be obtained from food and supplements. Essential nutrients must be obtained from food sources, because the body either does not produce them or produces them in amounts too small to maintain growth and health.

Your diet plan should allow for food that is most conducive to support your type of metabolism and balance your body chemistry. Try to eat the right foods as much as possible. You do not have to think in terms of calories. You should eat when you are hungry. In fact skipping meals is not a good idea because your body might think you're starving it. When this happens your body's self-preservation mechanism might kick in, which can lower your body's set point, thereby slowing down your metabolic rate, resulting in an increased tendency of your body to store food intake as fat instead of burning it up for energy. Think of your fuel mix (your food) for your engine of metabolism (your cells). The right fuel mix can provide you with the optimum energy production from your food intake. The wrong fuel mix can result in lower energy production, suboptimal performance, and a decreased sense of well-being. The autonomic system controls all involuntary activity in the body—digestion, elimination, heartbeat, and immune activity, for example—and is comprised of two divisions: sympathetic and parasympathetic, which allow for homeostasis of organs and basic physiological functions. In general, the parasympathetic nervous system is involved with digestion and energy, while the sympathetic nervous system is involved with energy expenditure and the fight-or-flight response. Our oxidative system is concerned with the rate at which nutrients are converted to energy in the cells through a process called oxidization.

The endocrine system exerts its influence on cellular metabolism through the secretion of hormones, which regulate various activities in the body. Genetically, each person has inherited various strengths and weaknesses in each of these systems. These variances provide the basis for all physiological and diet-related characteristics.

Each individual nutrient can have a more pronounced parasympathetic or sympathetic influence effect: either that of fast or slow oxidization or that of triggering a particular gland. The key to determining a well-balanced diet or supplement plan is to identify a metabolic balance for the general strengths and weaknesses of your autonomic nervous systems, your oxidative system, and your endocrine glands and then to eat foods and supplements that are designed to support your strength while strengthening your weakness. This helps balance the body's energy-producing systems, which promotes homeostasis and a state of optimal cellular balance. Your diet is far more important and powerful than supplements. Supplements should, and in reality do, "supplement" your diet. If you eat the right foods for your type and take the right supplements for you, you will have a potentially powerful combination for positively impacting your health and wellness.

Dietary proteins are powerful compounds that build and repair body tissues from hair and fingers to muscles. In addition to maintaining the body's structure, proteins speed up chemical reactions in the body, serve as chemical messenger molecules to assist the immune system to fight infection, etc., and transfer oxygen from the lungs to the body's tissues. Although protein provides four calories of energy per gram, the body uses protein for energy only if carbohydrate and fat intake are insufficient. When topped as an energy source, protein is diverted from the many critical functions it performs for our bodies. Proteins are made of small units called amino acids. Of the more than twenty amino acids, our bodies require eight (nine in young children). These amino acids cannot be made by the body in sufficient quantities to maintain health. They are considered essential amino acids and must be obtained from food. When we eat food high in proteins, the digestive enzymes break this dietary protein into amino acids, absorb them into the bloodstream, and send them to the cells that need them. Amino acids then recombine into the functional proteins our bodies need for protection.

Animal proteins found in such food as eggs, milk, meat, fish, and poultry are considered complete proteins because they contain all the essential amino acids our bodies need. Plant proteins are found in vegetables, grains, and beans, legumes; they lack one or more of the essential amino acids. However, plant proteins can be combined in the diet to provide all of the essential amino acids. A good example is rice and beans. Each of these foods lack one or more essential amino acids missing in rice and found in beans and vice versa. So when eaten together, these food provide a complete source of protein. Therefore vegetarians can meet their protein needs with diets rich in grains, dried peas and beans, rice, nuts, and tofu and soybean products.

Deficiencies in protein consumption may result in health problems. Marasmus and Kwashiorkor, both life-threatening conditions, are the most common forms of protein malnutrition. Fats, which provide nine calories of energy per gram, are the most concentrated of the energy-producing nutrients. Fats play an important role in building the membranes that surround our cells and in helping blood to clot.

Once fat is digested and absorbed, it helps the body to absorb certain vitamins. Fat stored in the body cushions vital organs and protects us from extreme cold and heat. If the body is deprived of essential fats it is subjected to losing its chemical balance.

Fats consist of fatty acids attached to a substance called glycerol. There are two essential fatty acids the body needs. The body cannot make them. Dietary fats are classified as saturated, monounsaturated, and polyunsaturated according to the structure of their fatty acids. Animal fats from eggs, dairy products, and meats are high in saturated fats and cholesterol, a chemical substance found in animal fat. Vegetable fats found in avocadoes, olives, some nuts, and certain vegetables are rich in monounsaturated and polyunsaturated fat. High intake of saturated fat can be unhealthy. Saturated fat is linked to high levels of cholesterol in the blood and development of heart disease, stroke, and other health problems. Despite its bad reputation, our bodies need cholesterol. Cholesterol is a "Protein" which is used to build cell membrane, to protect nerve fibers, and to produce vitamin D and some hormone chemical messengers that help coordinate the body's functions. Our liver, and to a lesser extent the small intestine, manufacture most of the cholesterol (Low-Density Lipo Protein) our body requires. Only about 20 percent is supplied from food.

Carbohydrates are the human body's key source of energy, providing four calories of energy per gram. When carbohydrates are broken down by the body, sugar (glucose) is produced. Glucose is critical to help maintain tissue protein, metabolize fat, and fuel the central nervous system.

Glucose is absorbed into the bloodstream through the intestinal wall. Some of this glucose goes straight to work in our brain cells and red blood cells while the rest makes its way to the liver and muscles, where it is stored as glycogen (animal starch or sugar), and to fat cells, where it is stored as fat. Glycogen is the body's auxiliary energy source, topped and converted back to glucose when we need more energy. Although stored fat can also serve as a back-up source of energy, it is never converted into glucose. Fructose and maltose, other sugar products resulting from breakdown of carbohydrates, go straight to the liver where they are converted into glucose.

Starches and sugars are the major carbohydrates. Common starch foods include whole-grain breads and cereals, pasta, corn, beans, peas, and potatoes. Naturally occurring sugars are found in fruits and many vegetables; milk products; and honey, maple sugar, and sugar cane. Foods that contain starches and naturally occurring sugars are referred to as complex carbohydrates because their molecular complexity requires our bodies to break them down into simpler form to obtain the much-needed fuel, glucose. Our bodies digest and absorb complex carbohydrates at a rate that helps maintain the healthful levels of glucose already in the blood.

In contrast, simple sugars refined from naturally occurring sugar added to processed foods require little digestion and are quickly absorbed by the body, triggering an unhealthy chain of events. The body's rapid absorption of simple sugar elevates the levels of glucose in the blood, which triggers the release of the hormone insulin. Insulin reins in the body's rising glucose levels, but at a price. Glucose levels may fall so low within one to two hours after eating foods high in simple sugars, such as candy, that the body responds by releasing chemicals known as anti-insulin hormones. This surge in chemicals, the aftermath of eating candy bars, can leave a person feeling irritable and nervous. Many processed foods not only contain high levels of added simple sugars, but they also tend to be high in fat and lacking in vitamins and minerals found naturally in complex carbohydrates. These processed junk foods provide only empty calories. They are depleted of nutrients, and many of them are carcinogens.

Some complex carbohydrates contain indigestible dietary fibers. Although such fibers provide no energy or building materials, they play a vital role in our health. Dietary fibers found only in plants are classified as soluble or insoluble. Soluble fibers found in such food as oats, barley, beans, peas, apples, strawberries, and citrus fruits will mix with food in the stomach and prevent or reduce the absorption by the small intestine of potentially dangerous substances from food.

Insoluble fiber found in vegetables, whole-grain products, and bran provides roughage that speeds the elimination of feces, which decreases the time that the body is exposed to harmful substance, which in turn reduces the risk of colon cancer. Studies of populations with low-fat and high-fiber-rich diets such as Africans and Asians show that these populations have less risk of colon and prostate cancer compared to those who eat low-fiber diets, such as North Americans.

Both vitamins and minerals are needed by the body in various amounts to trigger the thousands of chemical reactions necessary to maintain good health. Many of these chemical reactions are linked, with one triggering another. If there is a missing or deficient vitamin or mineral or link anywhere in this chain, this process may break down, with potentially devastating health effects. Although similar in supporting critical functions in the human body, vitamins and minerals have key differences.

Although they have many functions, vitamins enhance the body's use of carbohydrates, proteins, and fats. They are critical in the formation of blood cells, hormones, nervous system chemicals known as neurotransmitters, and the genetic material deoxyribonucleic acid (DNA). Vitamins are classified into two groups: fat soluble and water soluble. Fat-soluble vitamins, which include the vitamins A, D, E, and K, are usually absorbed with the help of foods that contain fat. Fat containing these vitamins is broken down by bile, a liquid released by the liver, and the body then absorbs the breakdown products and vitamins. Excess amounts of fat-soluble vitamins are stored in the body's fat, liver, and kidneys.

Water-soluble vitamins, which include vitamin C (ascorbic acid), B1 (thiamine), B2 (riboflavin), B3 (niacin), B6, B12, and folic acid, cannot be stored and rapidly leave the body in urine if taken in greater quantities than the body can use. Foods containing water-soluble vitamins need to be eaten daily to replenish body's needs. But some foods are better source of specific vitamin and minerals than others. For example, oranges contain large amounts of vitamin C and folic acid but little of the other vitamins. Milk contains large amounts of calcium but no vitamin C. I mention milk because most people in North America drink milk (I do not believe in drinking milk; milk is suitable only for baby cows). Sweet potatoes are rich in vitamin A, but white potatoes contain almost none of this vitamin. Because of these differences in vitamin and mineral content, it is wise to eat a wide variety of foods. Also, because of the conditions under which our foods are grown, transported, and processed, many of the essential nutrients are limited. Therefore, we need to supplement our diets to make up for the loss.

Whenever the body is not given enough of any one of the essential nutrients over a period of time, it becomes weak and less able to protect itself against pathogens and infections that attack the mind/body. The nervous, endocrine, digestive, immune, and other systems may be compromised, become sluggish, and react slowly in performing their duties to protect and heal the mind/body. Because of the lack of essential nutrients from the food, the mind/body will top its stored fat for energy, and muscle is broken down to use for energy. Eventually the body will not be able to defend itself and will become subjected to deficiency-related malnutrition.

Although malnutrition is more commonly associated with dietary deficiencies, it also can develop in cases where people have enough food to eat, but choose foods low in essential nutrients. This is a common form of malnutrition in developed countries such as North America. When poor food choices are made, a person may be getting an adequate or excessive amount of calories each day, yet still be undernourished, "well-fed, and starving."

In addition, vitamins A (in the form of beta-carotene), C, and E function as antioxidants, which are vital in countering the potential harm of chemicals known as free radicals. If these chemicals remain unchecked they can also transform chemicals in the body into cancer-causing agents. Environmental pollutants, such as cigarette smoke, are sources of free radicals.

Minerals are minute amounts of metallic elements that are vital for the healthy growth of teeth, bones, muscles, etc. They also help in such cellular activity as enzyme action, muscle contraction, nerve reaction, and blood clotting. Mineral nutrients are classified as major elements (calcium, chlorine, magnesium, phosphorus, potassium, sodium, and sulphur) and trace elements (chromium, copper, fluoride, iodine, iron, selenium, and zinc, etc.).

Vitamins and minerals not only help the mind/body perform its various functions but also prevent the onset of many disorders. For example, vitamin C is important in maintaining our bones and teeth; scurvy, a disorder that attacks the gums, skin, and muscles, occurs when this substance is missing. Diets lacking vitamin B1, which supports neuromuscular function, can result in beriberi, a disease characterized by mental confusion, muscle weakness, and inflammation of the heart. Adequate intake of folic acid by pregnant women is crucial to avoid nervous system defects in the developing fetus. The mineral calcium plays a critical role in building and maintaining strong bones; without it children develop weak bones and adults experience the progressive loss of bone mass known as osteoporosis, which increases their risk of bone fractures.

When the body is not given enough of any one of the essential nutrients over a period of time, it becomes weak and less able to fight infection. The brain may become sluggish and react slowly. The body taps its stored fat for energy, and muscle is broken down to use for energy. Eventually the body withers away, the heart ceases to pump properly, and death could occur, the most extreme result of the dietary condition known as deficiency-related malnutrition.

In addition to vitamins and minerals, there are plant substances, which are called phytochemicals. Phytochemicals are naturally occurring biochemicals that give plants their color, flavor, smell, and texture. There is increasing evidence that phytochemicals may help prevent many of the degenerative diseases that culminate in an exceptionally high death rate from heart disease, cancer and strokes. These are responsible for over 60 percent of all deaths in the United States. Some phytochemicals such as digitalis and quinine have been used for medical purposes for centuries. The anti-cancer effects of many of these plant substances are only now beginning to be investigated. Phytochemicals differ from vitamins and minerals in that they have no known direct nutritional value. Some are antioxidants, protecting agents against harmful cell damage from cellular oxidization. Others perform different functions that help prevent cancer. Today's food scientists are still identifying the beneficial substances and deciphering the many ways phytochemicals in foods offer frontline defenses against cancer and other diseases. There are hundreds, perhaps thousands, of these protective substances in food and plants. Fruits and vegetables are considered to be the best sources. During the past century, medical science has added wondrous treatments and technologies to its disease-fighting arsenal. For all these innovations, however, the most amazing and effective weapon for fighting cancer and other disease are found in our plant-based foods.

Available research from over 200 studies of human populations from around the world has identified fresh (vine-ripened) fruits and vegetables as the most beneficial source of phytochemicals. Five to ten servings daily are recommended. The average American or Canadian eats about four serving per day. Nutrition and medical science are continuing to identify and study new phytochemicals. Daily use of these protective substances is considered the best healing therapy for mind/body.

Carbohydrates have always been considered as energy food, but not until 1994 was it discovered and in 1996 proven and recognized in Harper's biochemistry textbook that there are eight monosaccharides (sugar carbs) essential to maintaining good health. The efficiency of these sugars, also knowing also as glyconutrients, has been established by the world's leading scientists and researchers as the key to proper cellular communication and proper cell function. It is suggested by some researchers that their "surface sugar" can inhibit tumor growth. Glyconutrients are the key to unlocking all chemical reaction of life-giving energy. They are the fundamental basis of effective healing systems. These substances, which form an integral part of the condition of normality or optimum health, are considered an essential factor in optimum health. These substances are referred to as "nutrients." Without a thorough understanding of precisely what it is that constitutes this condition of normal or optimum health it is not possible to fully understand any deviation from this condition. Neither is it possible to deliberately restore or maintain normality or optimum functioning of the mind/body.

Science teaches us that it is within the cells and mitochondria that the countless chemical reactions occur that determine our health and well-being. It is here also that the nutrients are required in optimum amounts. To attempt to treat any illness with foreign chemicals without first addressing any deviation in proper cellular nutrient levels represents not a departure from science but a total departure from basic common sense. In keeping with these facts we must also acknowledge the frailty of attempting to assess nutritional status by measuring nutritional levels and the blood as if this is some kind of guarantee that nutrients will therefore be constantly delivered to all the billions of cells in the body in optimum amounts.

To continue with carbohydrates, there is a scientific knowledge that provides healing for every cell in our bodies, eliminates our diseases, prevents malfunctions, and repairs our body's internal structure. This can be done with nature's natural formula, which was given to man by our Creator and is just now being discovered by some of our world's leading scientists and dedicated physicians, who have heard the public cry for help.

Hippocrates, the father of medicine, and many other preventative-medicine physicians and nutritional researchers have been sounding the nutritional and biochemical symphony of truth and hope for suffering humanity to be free from degenerative diseases caused by the likes of environmental poisons, man-made chemicals, toxic wastes, polluted water, processed and refined foods, nutritional deficiency of foods and emotional stressors which cause misery,, pain and death.

My sadness for millions of people (and I include myself here) who have lived in pain, fear and suffering of mental, spiritual, physical, and emotional frustration, can be relieved by this new scientific discovery, which deals with chemical molecules that can help the cells of our body communicate effectively with each other and provide a more efficient defense against infectious diseases and repair damages caused by pathogens and free radicals. In order for us to live healthy lives we must have these molecules in our bloodstream and cells. Our body can make some of these messenger molecules, but it needs the raw materials, which come from plants and minerals. These plants and minerals create a process that has been designed from the beginning of creation to protect and heal us daily. God, through his divine wisdom, has created all the necessary nutritional factors in nature to provide for our everyday healing. If we provide the body with what it needs, the body will take care of itself.

Nutritional science only suspected that these molecules existed, but recently with the help of advanced biochemical techniques we now know precisely what these molecules are, what they do, how they are made, and how we can get them. Now we acknowledge that the reason for eating is to get these specific nutrients in our body. In the early days of scientific medical discovery the field of biochemistry explored the inner secret of food in an effort to discover what was in food that gives us life. Carbohydrates, fat, and protein were thought to be the essentials of life.

As knowledge increased, we found essential ingredients in products that are the life-giving substances that are called amino acids. Someone else discovered that there are certain amino acids that we must get from the food we eat because our bodies cannot make them. They are called essential amino acids. Then science discovered that there are essential ingredients in the general category of fats that we must get from the food we eat because our bodies cannot make them. They are called fatty acids. And now we know that there are essential fatty acids.

Scientists used to think that carbohydrates were simply various forms of sugar molecules and that their primary purpose was to provide fuel energy for the working of our bodies. The latest breakthrough discovery is that there are certain carbohydrate molecules that are chemical messengers, not a source of energy. These messenger molecules are what actually enable the cells of our body to function normally.

These non-starch polysaccharides are long-chain carbohydrates, or sugar, which in past generations was once more common in human food, but has been processed out or excluded it from the modern diet. Scientists have discovered that there are eight separate and distinct carbohydrate molecules needed, and only one or two of them are coming into our bodies through the modern food we eat. This means that cells are not receiving the vital instruction they need, and therefore they malfunction. When these malfunctions accumulate as signs and symptoms of diseases, certain combinations of the messenger molecules are necessary for proper internal function. If there is deficiency, cancer and other degenerative diseases are the result.

Research studies published in the *Journal of Glycobiology* have shown that our cells selectively pull these saccharides from our blood when available. These findings provide direct evidence that our cells are not designed for cellular conversions of glucose (a back-up system) to supply the essential saccharides. In an article titled "Capitalizing on Carbohydrates" by Jon Hodgson in the *Journal of Bio/Technology*, Vol. 8 Feb. 1990, it states, "Almost without exception, whenever two or more living cells interact in specific ways, cell surface carbohydrates will be involved."

Tens of thousands of people who have suffered from chronic disabling diseases have visited their doctors. They get painkillers like drugs, stimulants etc. Most of them don't get better unless they heal themselves, and many times they get worse if they can't heal themselves. Why can't the drugs work in these cases? Because it is not the lack of drugs that causes the problems. The problems come about as a result of deficiencies in the body's internal chemistry.

As nutritional science advanced, additional nutrients were discovered. Vitamins, minerals, and enzymes came to our awareness. Medical science believes that we get all the vitamins and minerals by eating three square meals a day. I am afraid that will not work. Nutritional science knows that we need to supplement our diet with essential supplements of vitamins, minerals, and enzymes. And now we are beginning to realize that the vitamins and minerals will work more effectively with the eight essential saccharides molecules.

The important question is, what are these saccharides molecules, upon which our health depends, and where can we get them? Only two of the essential monosaccharides—glucose from sweet foods and carbohydrates, and galactose from dairy products—are found in our diet today! Why? During the past twenty-five years, our food supply has changed from home gardens and local farms that provided vine-ripened fruits and vegetables to such industrialization that now almost all fruits and vegetables are grown on large commercial farms. The soil on these farms is depleted of nutrients and minerals. The soil is sprayed with toxic chemicals to kill weeds and insects and fertilized with nitrogen, potassium, and phosphorous, which still makes plant grow, but lacks vital trace minerals. Then to add to all the other negatives, produce is harvested green so that it can be transported across the country or ocean and withstand shipment. The produce is not allowed to ripen on the vine. Our fruits and vegetables do not have all the phytochemicals that the American Cancer Society says are so important to building our immune system. Phytochemicals are produced in our plants only when they are fully vine-ripened.

We further deplete our grains, source of some essential sugars, by hauling and removing the germinal portions of wheat, rice, oats, etc. The result of this is that six of the eight essential monosaccharides are no longer in our diet. We also deteriorate our food by processing methods, preservatives, and over-cooking. Fortunately, our body can make the missing six carbs (glycoprotein) by a complicated, energy-consuming process using fifteen or more reactions, each requiring a specific enzyme—if everything is working perfectly. Obviously, everything is not always working perfectly or there would be no health problems. The most important essential to health and quality life is missing.

There are more than 200 monosaccharides in nature. These are simple sugar molecules. We now know that eight of these molecules combined with protein and lipid are used by our body to make the messenger molecules call glycoprotein. As stated before, carbohydrates have always been considered as energy food, but not until 1994 was it discovered, and in 1996 proven and recognized in Harper's biochemistry textbook, that there are eight monosaccharides (carbohydrates) essential to maintaining good health.

These eight carbohydrate-protein combinations (glycoprotein or glyconutrient) make the messengers that conduct our defense against infections and repair our damaged cells. Glyconutrients are plants, carbohydrates (monosaccharides), and biologically essential plant sugars. Galactose, glucose, fructose, mannose, zylose, N-acetylglocosamine, N-acetyl-galactosamine, and N-acetyl-neuramic-acid are some examples. Typical of these are interleukins, prostaglandins, leukotrenes, tumor necrosis factors, and colony-stimulating factors. These are molecules that enable our cells to communicate with others. When cells become cancerous they do so because of defective communication of cells. When the body attempts to correct the problem and destroy the tumor, the messenger molecules work as negotiators between the life and death of us or the cancer or other diseases.

Most of the monosaccharide building blocks that are in our diet are sugars known as fructose sucrose. They comprise the bulk of our carbohydrates, but those are not the essential saccharide molecules that are the subject of discovery. They are part of those that can be used by the body to construct the essential carbohydrates or saccharides, which can then be used entirely or in part to build the glycoproteins that are among the more important cell-to-cell messengers and receptors. If we do no get the essential saccharides molecules in our diet or in supplements form, our bodies are forced to manufacture them from scratch, which the body can do. But there are three problems in this manufacturing, and it is from these problems that most diseases originate and many diseases can be cured.

The first problem is that production of these components requires a great amount of energy, which the body must take from other vital functions. The second problem is that under the best of conditions the body chemistry cannot make enough of these messenger molecules by building them from scratch. The third reason is that each of the many steps of manufacturing the glycoprotein molecules requires specific gene instruction, enzymes, and supervision. The genes themselves may be defective or in a state of disrepair. Therefore the choice and responsibility is yours and mine to provide our body with the right combination of food and supplements.

The question is why these glycoproteins are so smart. Glycoproteins are smart because they are not drugs, which act no matter if they are needed or not. The practitioner prescribing them has to pay close attention to dose. Let's say my wife has high blood pressure. When her doctor prescribes drugs she has to prescribe the right dose. The wrong dose can drop the blood pressure too much, which is even worse than high blood pressure in some cases. However glycoproteins are simply supplements (carbohydrates and protein). They replace what the body needs and no more. In some cases large doses of glycoprotein must be taken because of more severe disease states and of poor absorption and utilization of sugar, but you cannot overdose on glycoprotein, because an excess of supplements will be ignored by the body because it is not needed and will simply be flushed out of the system.

Glyconutrients increase natural killer-cell function. This result protects healthy individuals from the effects of toxins and free radicals, which could cause infections and cancer formation. In chronic diseases with decreased functions, the activity is tremendously increased, leading to improvement of the disorder. Furthermore, glycoproteins increase T-cell function and decrease abnormally elevated apoptosis without disturbing the normal balance in the body. Glycoprotein is ideal and safe for immune system protection, while assisting us with diseases associated with immune suppression, including cancer and other diseases. Your immune system is the best medicine you have. If you give it the proper tools, it will very likely be able to protect you from any problem and provide optimal health and wellness.

These complexes, polysaccharide dietary supplements, contain most or all of the eight essential saccharides. They are obtained from various sources, including rice, barley and bran, mushrooms, yeast cell walls, aloe vera, and gum sugars. The more essential saccharides you add to your diet, the fewer number of steps, enzymes, and energy the body expends processing them for us. Most healthy people can generate every other essential saccharide from glucose. But if the person is sick or stressed out, the body may not be able to marshal the resources it needs to convert one sugar to another. Supplying all eight essential saccharides takes the burden off an overstressed body.

Researchers know that cancer is a cellular disease, but they are not willing to allow the natural process of the body's internal metabolism to do its work. It is a known fact that if you provide the body with all the essential factors it will do its work. Cellular medicine is a positive solution to cancer. The cardiovascular system is one of the most active of our mind/body and has the highest consumption of essential nutrients. Our endothelial cells (blood vessel wall cells) form the protective layer between blood and blood vessel wall. These cells contribute to a variety of metabolic functions such as optimum metabolic blood viscosity. The smooth muscle cells produce collagen and other reinforcement molecules to provide optimum stability, reinforcement, and tone to the blood vessel walls.

Blood Cells

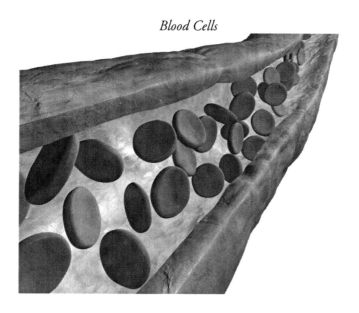

Blood cells are the pipelines of the mind/body; measuring 60,000 miles, they supply life-saving nutrients to the body, including the millions of blood corpuscles circulating in the blood stream. They are responsible for oxygen transport, defense, scavenging, wound healing, and many other functions. The deficiency in essential macro and micronutrients in the different cell types is closely associated with most cellular diseases plaguing our society, due to exposure to all the environmental pollutions and toxin. Long-term deficiency of these essential nutrients in millions of vascular wall cells impairs the function of blood vessel walls.

Cancer cell stuck in small capillary wall of cell

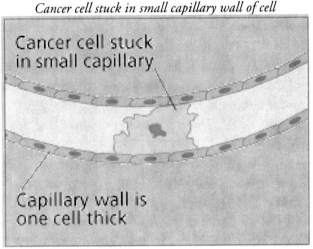

"Taken from CancerHelp UK"

Cell biologists are concentrating on cell membrane in the immune system and all cells in the body. This is where all the cell communication takes place, and this is where mutation takes place. Since early proposal of Boverin more than a century ago, multiple experimental evidence has confirmed that, at the molecular level, cancer is due to lesions in the cellular-level DNA. First it was observed that a cancer cell transmits to its daughter cells the phenotypic features characterizing the cancerous state. Second, most of the recognized mutagenic compounds are also carcinogenic, having as a target cellular DNA. Finally, the karyotyping of several types of human tumors, particularly those belonging to the hematopoietic system, lead to the identification of recurrent quantitative and numerical chromosomal aberrations, reflecting pathologic re-arrangements of cellular genome. When taken together, these observations suggest that the molecular pathogenesis of human cancer is due to structural alterations of specific genes whose function is to control cellular growth and differentiation. There are about 100,000 genes in the chromosomes of each cell. The genes are carried in the DNA and are the blueprint of all the characteristics that were inherited from the parents. Studies have indicated that a few of these genes, about 100, are oncogenes, genes that can cause cancer. The cells of our body normally reproduce or split exactly in half when it is necessary to replace or repair cells or tissues. Some studies suggested that when oncogenes are "hit" by carcinogens, they reproduce, resulting in new cells that may be abnormal cells.

Since the turn of the century, researchers have been searching for this specific gene that mutates and causes cancer. There are several reports that suggested that they have found a gene that might be the cause of prostate cancer; however, the reports always concluded with the same statement: More study is needed.

The good news is that there are nutritional natural foods and supplements available to protect and repair cellular damage. The origins of cellular disease can be considered from two cellular aspects—the lack of biological fuel needed by the cells' mitochondria or a failure in the function of the metabolic control center of the cell.

Deficiency of specific essential nutrients, environmental pollutions, and toxin damage to cellular DNA contribute to the development of cancer in the body at the cellular level. Damage to the cellular DNA destroys the control mechanism of cells' replication, which allows abnormal cells to continuously grow in the body during one's lifetime. "New" cells are surrounded by collagen and connective tissue, which provide support for the human body. For healthy cells to expand and grow, they have to break down the extracellular barrier that confines them. This process is essential for life of all human, and for this reason cells need to produce and secrete enzymes that digest connective tissue components, including collagen and elastin. It is important that these enzymes be regulated with precision so that the integrity of the connective tissue and its supports are never compromised, because excessive disintegration of connective tissue can cause pathology.

Cell biologists are now concentrating on the cells in the body. This is where cell communication is performed and cells help other cells function and develop correctively, keeping good things in and bad things out and regulating the flow of substances in and out of the cells. And when essential chemicals are attached to the cells, proper immune functions protect the human body. In fact, without proper cell membrane functions, none of us would be here, because the sperm could not fertilize the egg in the embryo, or too many sperm would fertilize the egg. If this happens at the two-cell stage, the mind/body would not be able to decide which cell to form, because all cells in the body have the capacity to be any kind of cell. Only proper cell membrane communication can make the right cells for our tissues and organs. Cell-to-cell communication is the key that provides optimum health of mind/body.

Apoptosis, a term that refers to cell suicide, is an important factor in a cell's communication system. It is an important, normal process in the body's immune system. When cells are damaged by toxins or other mechanisms, especially damage to the DNA, the cell must decide between one of two options: to try and repair itself, or to commit suicide (apoptosis). Cells commit suicide because damaged cells have the potential to become cancerous. When cells grow out of control, they replace normal body tissue and produce toxic chemicals, which could lead to the death of the individual if left uncontrolled. The growth of uncontrolled cells is the cause of immune cells reprogramming themselves with the capability to attack the cells in your mind/body because of their inability to recognize which cell is self and which cell is foreign.

It is important to understand why this process of apoptosis is so critical to a healthy immune function of the human mind/body, because in several disease this process goes out of control and happens so easily, which leads to loss of immune cell capability and an unbalance or deficient immune system as the body tries to regulate and replace these cells; if the communication problem is not resolved, cancer or other self-destructive diseases will occur. Cell-surface glycoprotein vitamins and minerals and other essential factors are the key to aid the immune system in providing a cancer-free body. There is also a missing ingredient that is needed to allow our healing system to successfully provide spiritual and physical healing.

From the beginning of time, understanding the human mind-body has been a challenge to scientists, health care professionals and lay persons. With every new discovery comes a new mystery to be unraveled. Although we now have a much better understanding, of the human mind-body and its performance, there is an incredible amount of things we do not know or understand, and may never understand. Our desire and enthusiasm to learn more increases our quest to explore and solve the mysteries of life. Note, however, that all our good intentions can lead to more technology development while seeking out more useful information.

We are to be careful, however, that we do not ignore the benefits of the most important factors for real healing - that is, natural God-given foods.

Since the advancement of technology, the human body has become a source of fascination to satisfy human thirst for knowledge and fame. Every day there are new discoveries: new drugs, new procedures, new products, and new diets, to name just some. In my search for a coherent approach to nutrition, I came to the realization that there is an essential ingredient missing from our dietary system. The missing ingredient is our spiritual connection with our Creator. We are more than a body needing nutritional requirements for health and wealth. We are clothed in the elements of divine power, love and infinite affection.

Our mind-body is a sacred vessel fashioned by our Creator to carry the spark of life. Without the breath of life, we are nothing. We are just a lifeless collection of elements. It is within the spiritual connectiveness with our Creator that our life journey begins. The natural food we eat and the air we breath reminds us that we are mortal, earthbound creatures, hungry and in need of spiritual, mental, physical and emotional wholeness of mind-body, with a need to successfully enjoy our journey of life. It is within this intriguing concept of life that our problems begin. For beneath our nutritional theories, our eating habits and lifestyle, we have separated ourselves from the most essential factor of life, our Creator's love. Our commission is to love the Lord with all our heart and mind, and our neighbors as ourselves.

Our quest for survival of the fittest has short-circuited our potential ability to love and care for ourselves and others. Our connection circuits are corroded and broken by insecurity, fear, selfishness, prejudice, hate and other negative emotions, and short- circuited our potential energy flow of love. In the book Ministry of Healing, E. G. White links the sickness of body and mind to nearly all its failings and discontent. Attitude influences the physical condition. No one can hate his or her neighbor and not have stomach trouble. Anger can destroy the brain as much as any disease tears down the body. Anger is itself a disease. For many people, it's not what they eat that's the problem; it's what's eating them! Anger is the most notorious criminal of the body. If not removed from our system, it will become an emotional baggage that restricts the free flow of harmonious healing. The strain between the physical, mental and spiritual attributes of any individual finds expression not only in the brain itself, but in the autonomic nervous system. A spiritual value helps in curing disease, and could be health's greatest safeguard.

In an article published in Healthy Living, the author suggested that the frontal lobe, located in the cerebrum, is the crown of the brain. This is where communication between humanity and divinity takes place. It is also where our conscious and subconscious perceptions and beliefs are defined and our characters are developed. It is the seat of judgment, reasoning, intellect for the will and wishes of God. A damaged frontal lobe causes deterioration of character that could lead to a dangerous lifestyle. The frontal lobe is referred to as the control center of our entire brain. Spirituality, character, morality, and the will are the characteristics that give us our unique individuality and allow us to make choices that influence our lives. Therefore, a person with a damaged frontal lobe could lose the ability to communicate effectively with others. It is the frontal lobe that differentiates humans from the animal kingdom. Humans have the largest frontal lobe and are able to perform more complex functions. Animals have a smaller frontal lobe, which limits their ability to analyze information and make judgments based on new information. Because of these deficiencies, they rely on instinct for survival.

Crown of the brain

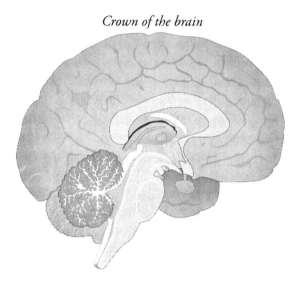

Humans should not depend on survival of the fittest to define their character. The frontal lobe is most likely where God communicates with us. If the frontal lobe is destroyed by a destructive lifestyle and environmental factors, our health will also be affected. We will be deficient of spiritual ability to communicate with our Creator. When the frontal lobe is constantly reprogrammed with negative thoughts and such suppressive information as elicit drugs and alcohol, it is like a computer virus. The virus will reprogram and damage our frontal lobe and brain cells, and diminish our capability and capacity to elevate spiritual reasoning. Learning ability will also be lessened. To maximize the full potential of our frontal lobe, it is imperative that we focus on the positive things of life: things that bring joy to ourselves and to others. We must avoid negative things that will compromise our healing system. When we practice love instead of hate, peace instead of war, acceptance instead of prejudice, faith instead of fear, giving instead of cheating, forgiveness instead of anger, we will defeat the enemy of selfishness, and allow our potential power of love to be reconnected to the divine source of love. It is within the sacredness of this spiritual realm that our journey of life continues with joy, no matter what negative situations we experience. "Let this mind be in you, which was also in Christ Jesus"

This missing important factor of divine love combined with a balanced nutritional program will provide an efficient, effective preventative maintenance program that will allow the body's incredible healing system to perform its infinite moment-by-moment healing of mind-body, and eliminate cancer cells and other diseases.

Chapter 8:
Conclusion

Data collected has shown that research related to nutrition and cancer is mega-funded internationally and concerns the identification of cancer-causing agents, the prevention of cancer by diet and nutritional supplementation, and protection from and treatment of cancer by individual nutrients or a combination of nutrients and with nutrients in combination with conventional chemotherapy and radiotherapy treatments. Research is carried out on many levels, ranging from large cohorts (30,000 people) in epidemiological studies to small-scale human clinical or case-controlled studies, a range of animal model studies, and at the biochemical and molecular level in cell-tissue lines. I will attempt to critically review the many facets of research on prevention and treatment of cancer and the massive amount of data, published by pre-eminent scientists in the most prestigious journals, which represent a massive amount of international effort over several decades. It is difficult to understand why doctors are not investigating and utilizing nutrition in the defense against the psychopathological and emotional epidemic of cancer in our Western society.

There is nothing more discouraging and frustrating to hopeful researchers and cancer patients than to learn of the courageous discoveries and innovations of pioneering and present scientists being thwarted by the attempts of established political and financial organizations to protect positions. It is even more frustrating to read lengthy, extensive documents describing battles against such scholarly innovators as

Nobel Laureate scientist Linus Pauling, and Roger Williams, Abram Hoffer, Carl C Pfeiffer, Dr Harry Alsleben...

It is suggested in the medical community that no one knows what causes some men to get prostate cancer while other men don't. Scientists and clinical researchers are working hard to discover the answer to this basic question. I am of the opinion that they are making this question more complicated by their overzealous enthusiasm to disprove the relevance of natural therapies or natural healing.

There are many hundreds of cancer trials being conducted in the United States, Canada, other countries. Most of these trials are sponsored by government agencies and pharmaceutical companies and are conducted at hospitals, cancer centers, and some doctor's offices. There is no single resource that lists all cancer trials. Many cancer centers, oncologists, and pharmaceutical companies have Web sites listing available clinical trials. The National Cancer Institute (NCI) has a comprehensive database of cancer research studies. This database includes information about finding ongoing trials, including nutritional research.

For over forty years, Judah Folkman, MD Professor of Cell Biology, has been researching anti-angiogenesis drugs to shut down the growth and migration of blood vessel cells to suppress the growth of tumor cells. In 1999, he had high expectations that his two anti-angiogenesis drugs, endostatin and angiostatin, were finally headed toward clinical trials. The ***New York Times*** suggested that Folkman's new drugs were the cure for cancers. His expectation was to have the drug work on people as it did on mice. But of course it was not so simple, and the result would not be known quickly. The question is what is an angiogenesis inhibitor?

An angiogenesis inhibitor is a naturally occurring or synthetic molecule that can interfere with or "block" angiogenesis (abnormal cell growth). Researchers are suggesting that because abnormal angiogenesis rarely turns itself off spontaneously, the goal of anti-angiogenesis therapy is to stop the formation of new blood vessels and to break up the existing abnormal blood vessels and not to affect normal resting blood vessels in the body.

However, if you read the full expectation, you will come to the conclusion that it is just another drug added to conventional medicine. Researchers are suggesting that angiogenesis inhibitors target the blood supply feeding the tumor, while surgery, standard chemotherapy, and radiation therapy target the tumor itself. They are predicting that eventually angiogenesis inhibitors may be added to chemotherapy or to radiation therapy or to other treatments such as vaccine therapy and gene therapy. Also, in the future, combinations of angiogenesis inhibitors may be used together. After forty years of research there are lots of unanswered questions.

Research conducted at the Center for Cancer Biology & Nutrition at Texas A&M University has discovered that tissues are comprised of a society of diverse cell types that must communicate to maintain normal function, peace, tranquility, and good health. They believe failure of cells to communicate properly underlies the cause of cancer and other degenerative diseases. Their laboratory studies of chemical signals (polypeptide growth factors and cytokines) in the local tissue environment control growth and specialization of different cell types of the prostate, the lungs, the vascular system, and the neural tissues. These chemical signals determine the normal development and function of the tissue while aberrations result in the tissue dysfunction and disease, such as cancer and other diseases, stroke, atherosclerosis, and liver and neural disease. They also suggested that the signaling systems, which is comprised of a signal polypeptide from one cell type and a reception system along with others, are the basis for communication among cells in tissue but also serve as sensors of signal-like hormones and nutrients that come from outside tissues. The cellular reception system for many signal polypeptides consists of a transmembrane protein whose external domain interacts with signal polypeptides and an intracellular domain that is a protein-kinase enzyme that activates metabolic pathways to control all cell-growth function and gene expression. The fibroblast growth factor (FGF) signaling system is an intrinsic tissue regulator that is the heart of homeostasis within adult tissues and in the embryogenesis.

"Mutation in mitochondrial DNA (mtDNA) plays an important role in the development of prostate cancer, according to research by scientists at Emory University School of Medicine and the University of California, Irvine."

The report stated that the mitochondrial DNA, which is separated from nuclear DNA, is found in hundreds of mitochondria located in the cytoplasm outside of each cell's nucleus. They suggested that some are also found within the chromosomes harboring the nuclear DNA. The mitochondria are often referred to as the powerhouse of the cell because they produce about 90 percent of the body's energy when the body is working at optimum efficiency.

Doctors and researchers at the Center for Molecular and Mitochondrial Medicine and Genetics at the University of California, Irvine, sequenced segments of mtDNA from isolated prostate cancer cells and found a variety of mutations including various mutations in the mtDNA cytochrome oxidase subunit (COI) gene. They then sequenced the COI gene in 260 prostate cancer tissue samples or blood cells from prostate cancer patients who had radical prostatectomies between 1995 and 2002 and fifty-four tissue samples from patients who had prostate biopsies and were found to be cancer free.

They found that 12 percent of all the prostate cancer samples had mutations in the COI gene, while less than 2 percent of the samples from patients found to be cancer free had mutations in this gene. A control sample of 1,019 individuals from the general population, 7.8 percent of individuals, had mutations in the COI gene. The researchers suggested that they found both germ-line (inherited) and somatic (acquired) mutation in the prostate cancer samples.

Doctors also suggested that because cytochrome oxidase subunit mutations are more common in individuals of African descent, scientists also analyzed a group of patients and controls of European ancestry. In this group they found the COI mutations in 11 percent of the prostate cancer specimens, 0 percent of the no-cancer group, and 6.5 percent in a general population sample of 898 Europeans.

To determine whether mtDNA mutations are causally related to prostate cancer, the researchers introduced into a prostate cell line mtDNA harboring a known disease-causing mtDNA mutation and, as a control, the same mtDNA but without the disease mutation. They injected the modified prostate cancer cells into mice to assess their tumor-forming ability. The prostate cancer cells with the mutant mtDNA generated tumors that were on average several times longer than the prostate cancer cells with normal mitochondria. The researchers concluded that the deleterious mtDNA mutation greatly enhanced prostate cancer growth.

Knowing all these facts, it is difficult to accept the suggestion that angiogenesis inhibitors made of synthetic molecule manufactured in the laboratory will block blood vessels transporting nutrients and oxygenated blood to tumor cells, and the good cells will not be affected by this process. Synthetic drugs, which in many instances are designed to mimic the natural process of biochemical operation of mind/body and known to produce side effects, do not discriminate. Drugs operate like guided missiles; they destroy everything in their range of fire - enemies and friends.

The ability to live a cancer-free life becomes the responsibility of the individual. Therefore, education is the key to healthcare. Drugs therapies are reserved for sickness-care programs. The ability of healthcare providers to provide extensive nutritional knowledge will lead to a health-conscious, responsible, motivated society that is willing to make educated lifestyle changes that include good nutritional habits.

Our new world order of the twenty-first century must be stimulated and supplemented with solid academic knowledge by government, healthcare providers, and our community.

There is a need to motivate members of the affluent society to combat their chronic intoxication of unhealthy habits and arrest their civilization-induced deficiency before they eventually, more or less seriously, become public burdens. A usable premise for active preventative maintenance is our only cure for degenerative diseases and is capable of eliminating an enormous amount of social and economic misery. Drugs are not the answer to our problems. Angiogenesis inhibitors (drugs) that are induced to block nutrients and oxygen from entering cancer cells could become more toxic to our system. The level of oxygenation is one of the fundamental, essential, and deepest important factors in the degree and function of brain cells to provide optimal mind/body performance and expression. Our lungs require the most expenditure of energy to enhance all the distribution of rich oxygenated blood and nutrients to all areas of the mind/body.

The amount of oxygen you can consume is called your "aerobic capacity." Thirty percent of the upgrade capacity comes from exercise activity, and 400 percent+ is possible through breathing techniques. Oxygen assists with elimination of toxins.

A clean body is more flexible if there is not enough oxygen for both the solidifying function and incomplete combustion to occur to excess. Leftover and incomplete combustion byproducts collect in cells, and the body becomes toxic or has a buildup of waste products, and disease weakens. When our body's oxygen level drops, cellular structure weakens. If our air supply oxygen is cut off, the waste products can't be burned, and the first reaction is brain damage; if continued for long we die. If the body's oxygen levels are maintained to adequate levels, the feeling of well-being can be continual.

Someone who usually has a buildup of waste products in their cells from low oxygen intake and eating of hydrogenated foods and is a short breather accumulates free radicals in his or her system. They are not getting enough oxygen, and the solidifying characteristics of hydrogen combined with free radicals have dominating effects to muscle, tissues, and organs, and bones become weak and brittle. When oxygen is replaced by hydrogen, waste and lactic acid in the muscle build up over time.

Body oxygen levels could drop for a variety of reasons, such as injury and disease. Air should have about 20 percent oxygen, but in cities it can drop to 10 percent, causing a reduction in ideal oxygenation, and we become poor oxygenators. Oxygen is primarily an electric/chemical process. For example, the cerebral spinal fluid serves as the medium for our brain and nervous system. Oxygen also supplies glucose, which is needed for the brain's ten billion or more nerve cells. The brain takes up at least 25 percent of the body's oxygen intake. It is also proven that cancer cells cannot survive in an optimum oxygenated body.

There are four other elimination organs that operate with the oxygenation system to eliminate waste, toxins, and other environmental factors from the mind/body to provide equilibrium and nutritional stability. We are in a cyclical, temporary stage of having minerals entering and leaving our bodies. We have an ongoing exchange of the old for the new, as part of us dies daily and part of us returns to life daily. New skin is made on the palm of our hands every twenty-four to forty-eight hours. We are being renewed all the time. The recycling places a demand on our mind/body. The uniqueness of our metabolic system will allow us to survive in any environment, but it pays the price and can be expensive.

One of the most fascinating advances of recent years is in the field of biochemical individuality. Roger J. Williams discovered the vitamin pantothenic acid. He also first concentrated and named folic acid and participated in pioneering research with other vitamins. Biochemical individuality is the key that unlocks the door to a holistic approach to preventative maintenance of the mind/body. Each human body is different in many respects, as different as our fingerprints, faces, and voices appear on the outside. Humans are genetically diverse, our internal and external metabolic type are unique, and all humans are different - physically, mentally, spiritually, and emotionally. Bodies differ in size, shape, and capabilities. Internal organs differ in size and capabilities. Digestion and absorption vary considerably in efficiency from person to person. Some people are allergic to or intolerant of common foods and become ill if they eat the foods that help others to achieve optimum health and wellness. Different environments and lifestyles demand different nutritional intake.

Nutritional requirements vary widely from person to person. Conventional nutrition assumes that all of us require the same amount of minerals, vitamins, and other dietary factors and assumes that all the nutrients we eat actually get into the cells' organs and tissues that need them. These oversimplifying assumptions are responsible for many failures to meet nutritional needs. To use nutrition and lifestyle changes as a method of preventative and therapeutic maintenance, it is imperative to keep clearly in mind that it is more important to know the person who has the illness than it is to know which illness the person has. All nutritional assessment must be tailored to the person's need.

To effectively prevent and eliminate prostate cancer, environmental factors have to take precedence over genetics, because even identical twins can have different expressions of their genes. Lack of nutrition can cause gross abnormality in growing embryos. Healthy foods, physical activity, and reduced stress are increasingly recognized as vital ingredients of cancer prevention and survival. All these findings are true, however, negating the fact that biochemical individuality must be taken into account by healthcare providers. It is a mistake to assume that what works well in a certain environment should necessarily be good worldwide. Modern health diets are very diverse. In one extreme, there is the high-protein, low-carbohydrate, high-fat diet. At another extreme are the low-protein, high-complex-carbohydrate, low-fat approaches.

Many diet promoters preach their particular program with religious conviction. They assume that because they personally have benefited from a particular nutritional program and have seen it work for others, theirs must be the only way for all humans. This philosophy is not necessarily true. Every successful nutritional program also has unsuccessful outcomes. "What is food for one man can be poison to another." All healthy nutrition programs, no matter how diverse, do have something in common. They tell you not to consume refined carbohydrates, tea, tobacco, white flour, white sugar, alcohol, etc. If you leave all of these things alone, you may likely feel better. However, if you are truly interested in optimizing your health, your weight, and your energy and avoiding cancer, degenerating diseases, and premature aging, one of the steps you should take is to educate yourself on the subject of biochemical individuality and metabolic process.

While genetics play a role in predisposing some people to cancer, other factors play a greater role. In fact, much of what appears to "run in the family" results from exposure to environmental factors, such as cancer-promoting chemicals or nutritional patterns and lifestyles. Many factors including diet, physical activity, viral and bacterial infections, radiation, exposure to carcinogens, sedentary lifestyle, polluted water, lack of sunlight, and stressors all influence one's risk of developing cancer.

In the past two decades researchers have revealed that emotional factors and lack of exercise can alter the body's resistance to cancer. Changing sedentary lifestyles, eating habits, and emotional states could play a powerful role in preventing or surviving this disease. Cancer begins with a major change in normal living cells. As stated previously, the transformation from a normal cell to a cancer cell is triggered by damage to DNA. Cancer is a disease that starts from the cellular level. The cell generally undergoes cellular division more rapidly than the cell from which it originates. The dangerous nature of cancer is the ability of abnormal cells to invade other organs and tissues and travel through the bloodstream and lymphatic system to other areas of the body, a process known as metastasis.

To conclude, the primary cause of prostate cancer and all other cancers may be a deficiency of certain nutrients from the diet and the body's inability to assimilate, digest, and absorb nutrients, eliminate waste, and allow the nervous, endocrine, cardiovascular, and immune systems to function at their potential. Detoxification is a necessary process to assist the cells, tissues, organs, and systems in the performance of their duties. The body's five elimination organs are designed to eliminate waste and all environmental toxins from the body. If they are not functioning at optimum efficiency, nutrition programs will not work, and the healing process will be compromised.

With all the advertising and marketing to get you to buy products from certain companies, it can sometimes get confusing. I will attempt to provide guidelines according to my research experience in nutrition. Only you can decide what is good for you.

Some foods digest more easily in the body. They are more convenient to use and give lots of energy and vitality. They are considered healing foods. They boost metabolism and provide complete nutrition. A general rule of thumb is that God, through nature, gives us exactly what we need to keep us healthy. If the food is processed and refined as many convenience foods are, healthy nutrients may be eliminated. Eating more natural and raw foods like those below will build and create a healthy mind-body.

A vegetarian diet is my choice. There are several studies suggesting that Seventh-day Adventist vegan vegetarians are healthier and live longer than non-vegetarians. However, to be a successful vegetarian, each person has to make his own decision based on good information and his individual need. To be a vegetarian, a person has to understand how to combine foods to receive the eight essential amino acids from protein. A balanced diet must contain protein, which provides eight essential amino acids. A balanced diet also requires two essential fatty acids, the right mix of vitamins and minerals, carbohydrates, fibers, and clean water, supported by exercise and proper breathing techniques. Your diet must be tailored to supply your individual, metabolic needs.

Life Begins at 65

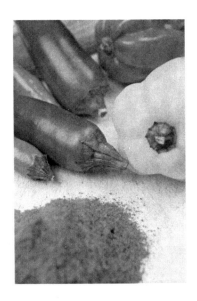

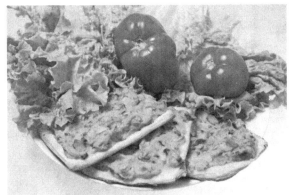

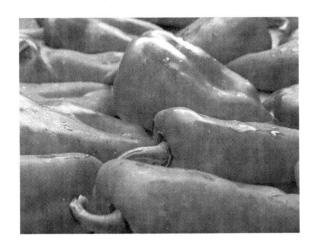

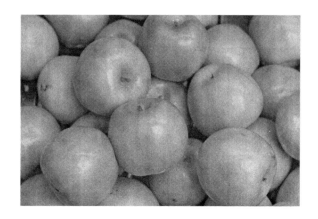

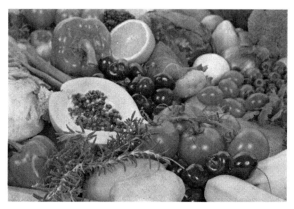

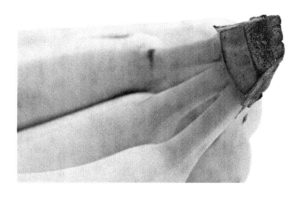

Life Begins at 65

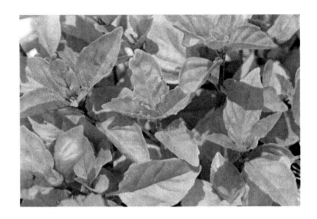

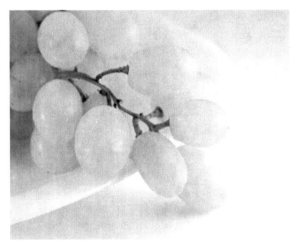

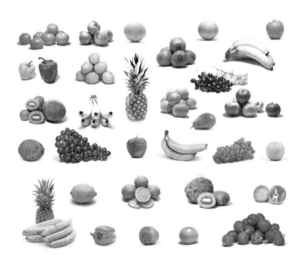

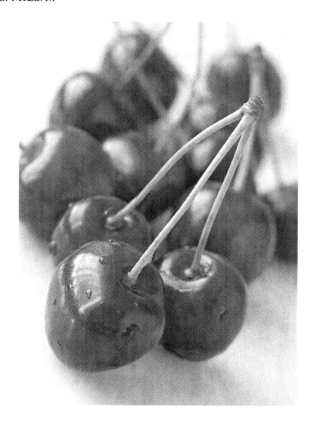

Fruits: Should be eaten first thing in the morning or for a nutritious late-evening snack. They will aid in cleaning out toxins. Choose from apples, pears, bananas, plums, cherries, apricots, nectarines, peaches, berries, currants, rhubarb, lemons, and clementines.

Vegetables: Always eat three times more vegetables than anything else. They are power-packed with vitamins and minerals (especially if they are organically grown and fresh). Vegetables can be eaten any time and can be eaten with either starch or protein. Choose from cabbage, broccoli, cauliflower, peppers, carrots, asparagus, cucumber, green and yellow beans, turnips, beets, snow peas, radishes, onions, Brussels sprouts, zucchini, mushrooms, bean sprouts, alfalfa sprouts, celery, leeks, kohlrabi, garlic, spinach, artichoke, eggplant, okra, tomato, endive, bok choy, parsley, and lettuce. Variety is the key to healthy eating. Most important are the green leafy vegetables, followed by the yellow, red, and orange varieties. White vegetables provide the least amount of nutrition.

Starches: (eat in moderation). Starches turn into sugar, and if not used as energy, e.g., through exercise, can be stored as fat. Many people with bowel problems will also find that if they limit starches they will have less problems. Some starchy vegetables are sweet potato, acorn squash, butternut squash, spaghetti squash, and pumpkin. Other starches come from potatoes, brown rice, basmati rice, whole grains, and corn.

Proteins: Too much animal protein can cause calcium to leach out of the body and create an acid pH. Try to substitute some of the good-quality vegetable proteins a couple of times per week: unfrosted/unsalted nuts and seeds - almonds, brazil nuts, pecans, hazelnuts, filberts, sunflower seeds, pumpkin seeds, sesame seeds, and pine nuts. Almonds are alkaline and therefore are beneficial in balancing pH. To make nuts more digestible, soak raw nuts in water overnight and throw out the soak water the following day. This method causes the nuts to begin to sprout, making them a live food packed with enzymes. Peanuts, cashews, and pistachios should be limited.

Bean family: Includes legumes, kidney beans, chickpeas, and lima, black, navy, roman, and white beans, and lentils (green lentils may be hard to digest). Soak overnight and throw out the soak water; then cook. Do not add salt while cooking, as this make them tough. You may want to soak them twice so that they are easier to digest.

Fish: Try scallops, salmon, halibut, orange roughy, haddock, mackerel, and then cod, bluefish, red snapper, sole, swordfish, and any deep cold-water ocean-going fish. Don't deep-fry them or you will negate their goodness.

Poultry and Dairy: Choose turkey, eggs, chicken, or some natural cheeses. The harder and whiter the cheese, the better. White cheddar, parmesan, Swiss, gouda, mozzarella, edam, jarlsberg, feta, havarti, or goat cheese may be consumed in moderate amounts if the body permits. Plain unsweetened, unpasteurized, unflavoured yogurt can be eaten, also used in place of sour cream. Do not use fruit-on-the-bottom or flavoured yogurt, as those containing preservatives, coloring, and sugar. Organic yogurt is preferable.

Fats: Avoid margarine or hydrogenated vegetable oils; use cold press virgin olive oil and butter only.

Spirulina is a whole-food vegetable protein that is easy to digest. Its total function is to produce protein, carbohydrates, vitamins, amino acids, and many other vital nutrients so important in human health.

Beverages: Drink at least eight to ten glasses of pure clean water each day. Herbal teas and 100 percent not-from-concentrate juices (both fruit and vegetable) may also be consumed. When we realized that every important function in our body requires water. We will understand how important water is to the human body. The mind-body needs water to keep us hydrated. Our bodies are made up of about 55 to 60 percent water. Water makes up 83 percent of our blood, 74 percent of our brain and 22 percent of our bones. Water regulates body temperature, remove waste from our bodies and cushions our joints… Perspiration is a natural cooling process, that takes place when the body is over-heated. In response over two million sweat glands excrete moisture (about 99 percent water). Lack of sufficient water in the body, could cause constipation. Chronic dehydration is the cause of many of our illnesses. The control centre for the sense of thirst, is located in the hypothalamus of the brain. This centre plays a major role in the regulation of total fluid volume. A decrease in fluid volume, or an increase in the concentration of body fluid stimulates the thirst centre, and thus cause us to drink water or other fluids. In a healthy person, the quantity of water consumed each day is about equal to the quantity lost. Many people drink far too much soda pops, coffee, alcohol and other concentrated beverages. Practice to drink more pure water.

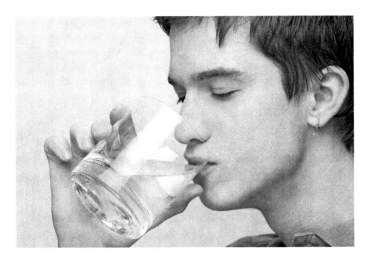

Your food choices have profound effects on your energy level, mood, sleep habits, and ability to cope with stress, and more. On the other hand, how you feel is intricately linked to what you choose to eat from one meal to the next. Poor eating habits establish patterns in the brain chemicals that regulate appetite and mood, which set you up for mood swings, food cravings, poor sleep habits, and other emotional problems that are not your personality and can contribute to health problems. The wrong combination of foods places undue stress on the digestive system. For example, fats inhibit and slow down the digestion of protein. Protein and sugar eaten together cause problems for our system. Sugar digests quickly in the stomach and small intestine. When eaten alone, they stay in your stomach for about 20 minutes. When they are eaten together with starches, proteins, and fats, they're delayed in our system, and become fermented.

Sprouts are an excellent source of Vitamin A, B, and E, such minerals as calcium, potassium, magnesium, iron and essential trace minerals: selenium and zinc. When sprouted, nature miraculously increases the total vitamin content, including Vitamin C, in each sprout. Your sprout can be harvested without losing any of their essential nutritional value. Sprouts and other raw foods are natural sources of antioxidants. Also, the best way to obtain food enzymes is to eat fresh raw fruits, vegetables and sprouted seeds. Cooking destroys food enzymes at about 105 degrees °F. Live food stimulates your metabolism and the regeneration process, supplies more bio-fuel to cells' power house (mitochondria) for efficient energy input and output.

What follows highlights some necessary nutrients and the results to your mind-body if these are lacking:

Calcium: If calcium is missing from the body, all minerals in the body are in delicate dynamic balance. Calcium metabolism and absorption requires adequate dietary magnesium, phosphorous and Vitamins A, C and D. Without these nutrients, it appears that calcium cannot be absorbed efficiently. Signs of deficiency include fragile, porous bones, heart problems, insomnia, muscle spasms, cramps and rickets.
Food sources of calcium are milk, milk products, sardines, turnips, mustard greens, broccoli, legumes, and dried fruits.

Chloride: Deficiency, infant loss of appetite, failure to thrive, weakness, lethargy, severe hypokalemia, metabolic acidosis.
Food sources: Seasalt, seafood, milk, meat and eggs.

Chromium: Deficiency, glucose intolerance, glucose and lipid metabolism abnormalities.
Food sources of chromium: Mushrooms, prunes, asparagus, organ meats, wholegrain bread, and cereals.

Copper: Deficiency, anemia, neutropenia, bone abnormalities.
Food sources of copper, liver, whole-grains, legumes, eggs, meat, fish.

Fluorine: Deficiency, dental caries, bone problems.
Food sources of fluorine, fish, meat, legumes, grains, legumes, drinking water (variable)

Iodine: Deficiency, enlarged thyroid gland, myxedema, cretinism, increase in blood lipids, liver gluconeogenesis, and extracellular retention.
Food sources of iodine: Iodized salt, salt water, seafood, sunflower seeds, mushrooms, liver, eggs.

Iron: Deficiency, listlessness, fatigue, anemia, palpitations, sore tongue, angular stomatitis, dysphagia, decreased resistance to infection.
Food sources of iron: Organ meats (liver), meat, molasses, nuts, legumes, seeds, green leafy vegetables, dried fruits, whole grains, cereals.

Magnesium: Deficiency, muscle cramps, kidney stones, heart attacks, atherosclerosis, disorientation and nervousness, epilepsy and faulty protein utilization. A prolonged deficiency causes the body to lose calcium and potassium, creating further deficiency in other metals involved in protein synthesis, weakness, tetany, abnormal behaviors, convulsions, growth failure.
Food sources of magnesium: nuts, legumes, cereals, grains, soybeans, parsnips, chocolate, molasses, corn, peas, carrots, seafood, brown rice.

Molybdenum: Defiance, hypermethioninemia, urinary xanthine, sulfite excretion, urinary sulfite and urate excretion.
Food sources of molybdenum: Soybeans, lentils, buckwheat, oats, rice, whole wheat bread.

Phosphorus: Deficiency, neuromuscular, skeletal and hematologist, renal manifestations, rickets, osteomalacia, anorexia.
Food sources of phosphorus: Meat, poultry, fish, eggs, milk, milk products, cereal grains, chocolate.

Sodium: Deficiency, anorexia, nausea, muscle atrophy, poor growth, weight loss.
Food sources of sodium: Sea salt, seafood, cheese, milk , bread, vegetables, (abundant in most food)

Sulphur: Deficiency, unknown
Food sources of sulphur: protein foods, meat, fish, eggs, milk, cheese, legumes, nuts

Selenium: Deficiency causes premature aging, liver malfunction, muscle atrophy
Food sources: Selenium is an essential trace mineral found in soil, water, plants and yeast. These naturally convert selenium into ergonomically

bound forms. Selenium works with vitamins C, E and other antioxidants in the body.

Zinc: Deficiency, poor wound healing, subnormal growth, anorexia, abnormal taste, smell, changes in hair, skin, nails, retarded reproductive system development.
Food sources of zinc: Wheat germ, beef, liver, poultry, whole grains.

Vitamin A: Deficiency causes cystitis, sinusitis, bronchitis, gastritis, loss of appetite, retarded growth, eye problems, night blindness, red eyes, bad vision, defective teeth, dry scaly skin, psoriasis, acne, wrinkles, pimples.
Food sources of Vitamin A fish and liver. Supplement with natural Beta Carotene to prevent risk of Vitamin A overdose. Source of Beta Carotene yellow-oranges, vegetable plants, leafy vegetables carrots, chili pepper and fish liver oil.

Vitamin C: Deficiency causes soft bleeding gums, decaying teeth, spontaneous bruising, lowered resistance to all infections and airborne poisons, skin hemorrhage, nose bleeds, anemia, toxic thyroid, premature aging, physical weakness, rapid breathing and heart beat, reduced adrenal secretions, tendency to ulcers of stomach and duodenal. Absence of Vitamin C causes scurvy.
Food source of Vitamin C: Citrus, rosehips, acerola berries, tomato, cabbage, fruit and vegetables in general.

Vitamin E: deficiency causes degeneration of coronary system, heart disease, strokes, pulmonary embolism, sterility, pains in the muscles, nerve system, eye and cerebral hemorrhage, dermatitis, enema, fragility of red blood cells.
Food sources, of vitamin E, vegetables and seeds oils, green leaves, and green leafy vegetables.

Vitamin K: Deficiency causes hemorrhaging anywhere in the body, premature aging and low energy.
Food sources of Vitamin K: Green leafy vegetables, egg yolk, cheese.

Vitamin D: Deficiency causes rickets, tooth decay, pyorrhea, osteomalacia, retarded growth, muscular weakness, low energy, lack of mineral and premature aging.
Food sources of Vitamin D: Fish liver oil, (eggs), sunlight.

Vitamin B1 (thiamin): Deficiency causes beriberi, muscle weakness, anorexia, tachycardia, enlarged heart and edema.
Food sources,of Vitamin B1: Seeds, nuts, wheat germ, legumes, lean meat.

Vitamin B2 (riboflavin): Deficiency causes cheilosis, glossitis, hyperemia and edemia of pharyngeal and oral mucous membrane, angular stomatities, photophobia.
Food sources of Vitamin B2: Non-fat milk, organ meat, egs, nuts, legumes, mushrooms, ricotta cheese.

Vitamin B3 (niacin): Deficiency causes pellagra, diarrhea, dermatitis, mental confusion or dementia.
Food sources of Vitamin B3: Meats, nuts, legumes, tuna, beef-liver, chicken breast, mushrooms.

Vitamin B6: Deficiency causes pernicious anemia, dermatitis, glossitis, convulsions.
Food sources of Vitamin B6: Meat and meat products which have derived their cobalamins from micro-organisms. All naturally occurring Vitamin B12 is produced by micro-organism, therefore micro-organism in the intestine could provide some source of B12.

Pantothenic acid: Deficiency very rare; numbness and tingling of hands and feet, vomiting, fatigue.
Food sources of pontothenic acid: Egg yolk, liver, kidney, yeast.

Biotin: Deficiency very rare; anorexia, nausea, glossitis, depression, dry scaly dermatitis.
Food sources of biotin: Synthesizied by micro-flora of digestive tract, yeast, liver and kidney.

Folic acids: Deficiency causes megaloblastic anemia, diarrhea, fatigue, depression, confusion.

Food sources of folic acid: Brewer's yeast, spinach, asparagus, turnip, greens, lima beans, beef liver.

Potassium, sodium, and chlorine are the three dominant electrolytes in the human body. Other electrolytes are magnesium, bicarbonate, phosphate, sulphur and proteins. Electrolytes are electrically charged atoms or molecules that conduct electricity as they dissolve in liquid such as blood or water. There are many electrolytes dissolved in blood, lymph, plasma, tissue fluids, and cellular fluids.

All of the above vitamins and minerals can be supplemented.

Glossary

Angiogenesis: The physiological process involving the growth of new blood vessels from pre-existing vessels. Angiogenesis is the term used for spontaneous blood-vessel formation, and intussusception is the term for new blood vessel formation by splitting of existing ones. Angiogenesis is a normal process in growth and development as well as in wound healing

Antigen: A substance, usually protein or protein-sugar complex in nature, which, being foreign to the bloodstream or tissues of an animal, stimulates the formation of specific blood serum antibodies and white blood cell activity. Re-exposure to similar antigens will reactivate the white blood cells and antibodies programmed against this specific antigen.

Apoptosis: Cells that are damaged by injury, such as by mechanical damage or exposure to toxic chemicals, undergo a characteristic series of changes; or cells that are induced to commit suicide.

Assimilation: The absorption of nutrients into the body after digestion in the intestine and transformation in biological tissues and fluids.

Benign: Literally innocent; not malignant. Often used to refer to cells that are not cancerous. They tend to grow slowly and don't spread (metastasize) like cancer tumors do.

Biopsy: Removal of a sample of tissue from a living being for diagnosis. A pathologist later uses a microscope to look for certain features, such as cancer cells, in the sample.

Brachytherapy: A relatively new procedure that involves implanting radioactive pellets into the prostate, where they gradually lose their radioactivity over a period of months. The pellets are inserted under general or spinal anesthetic.

Calcium: The body's most abundant mineral. Its primary function is to build and maintain bones and teeth. The body also needs calcium to carry nerve signals, keep the heart functioning, contract muscles, clot blood, maintain healthy skin, and help control blood acidity and alkaline balance.

Cancer: The various types of malignant neoplasms that contain cells growing out of control and invading adjacent tissues, which may metastasize to distant tissue.

Carcinogen: Any substance or agent that promotes cancer. Carcinogens may cause cancer by altering the metabolism or damaging DNA directly in cells, which interrupts normal biological processes.

Chemicals: Any material with a definite chemical composition, no matter where it comes from. For example, a sample of water has the same properties and the same ratio of hydrogen and oxygen whether the sample is isolated from a river or made in a laboratory. A pure substance cannot be separated into other substances by any mechanical process. Typical chemical substances found in the home are water, salt (sodium chloride), and sugar (sucrose). Generally, substances exist as solid, liquid, or gas and may change between these phases of matter with changes in temperature or pressure.

Chromogranin "A", Chromogranin "A" is a protein, located in neuroendocrine cells, which is co-secreted with a wide variety of peptide hormones and neurotransmitters.

Detoxification: The metabolic process by which toxic waste is removed from the human body.

Digestion: The process of metabolism whereby a biological entity processes a substance in order to chemically and mechanically convert the substance into nutrients.

Deoxyribonucleic Acid (DNA): A nucleic acid that contains the genetic instructions for the biological development of a cellular form of life or virus. All known cellular life and some viruses have DNA. DNA is a long polymer of nucleotides that encodes the sequence of amino acid in proteins, using the genetic code.

Gleason Grading: When the pathologist looks at the biopsy, he grades the cancer by comparing the appearance of the cancer cells to the appearance of normal prostate tissue. The grades go from Grade 1, almost normal, to Grade 5, very abnormal.

Elimination: The process of cleansing the body of waste and toxins. The colon and the kidneys are the primary elimination organs of the body. They eliminate waste and toxins from the body. If they are not functioning properly, there is a likely buildup of toxins in your body.

Endocrine System: Influences almost every cell, organ, and function of our bodies. It is instrumental in regulating mood, growth, and development. The glands of the endocrine system and the hormones they release influence almost every cell, organ, and function of your mind/body.

Enzymes: Specific protein catalysts produced by the cells that are crucial in chemical reactions and in building up and synthesizing most compounds in the body. Each enzyme performs a specific function without consuming itself.

Estrogen: One of the female sex hormones produced by the ovaries. While estrogens are present in both men and women, they are usually present at significantly higher levels in women of reproductive age. They promote the development of female secondary sex characteristics, such as breasts, and are also involved in the thickening of the endometrium and other aspects of regulating the menstrual cycle.

Genes: The units of heredity in living organisms. Genes are encoded in an organism's genome, are composed of DNA or RNA, and direct the physical development and behaviour of the organism. Most genes encode proteins, which are biological macromolecules comprising linear chains of amino acids that affect most of the chemical reactions carried out by the cells. Some genes do not encode proteins, but produce noncoding RNA molecules that play key roles in protein.

Genetics: The science of genes, heredity, and the variation of an organism. Heredity and variations form the basis of genetics. In modern research, genetics provide important tools for the investigation of the function of a particular gene.

Gland: Can be either a general tissue or an organ that secretes chemicals, and there are two types of gland—exocrine and endocrine. The glands that secrete chemicals through tubules or ducts are called exocrine and include sweat, tear, and salivary glands. Ductless glands secrete special chemical (hormones) directly into the bloodstream.

Herbs: Plants grown for culinary, medicinal, or in some cases even spiritual value. The green, leafy part of the plant is typically used. General usage differs between culinary herbs and medical herbs. A medicinal herb may be a shrub or other woody plant, whereas a culinary herb is a non-woody plant.

Hormones: Chemical substances secreted by a variety of body organs that are carried by the bloodstream and usually influence cells some distance from the source of production. Hormones signal some enzymes to perform their functions. They regulate body functions such as blood sugar levels, insulin levels, the menstrual cycle, and growth.

Immune System: Protects the body from infection by pathogenic organisms. It is composed of a complex constellation of cells, organs, and tissues, arranged in an elaborate and dynamic communications networks. The immune system is, in its simplest form, a cascade of detection and adaptation, culminating in a system that is remarkably effective.

Interferon: A protein formed by the cells of the immune system in the presence of a virus. It prevents viral reproduction and is capable of protecting non-infected cells from viral infections.

Journals: Published quarterly by associations of professors and experts from all parts of the world who have an interest in interdisciplinary research or in an effort to find meaning in our world. This association publishes studies dealing with those facts, things, ideas, persons, and values that people throughout history have considered ultimate and to which the human mind relates.

Karyotyping: Is a test to examine chromosomes in a sample of cells, which can help identify genetic problems, as in the case of disorder or disease. This test can

- Count the number of chromosomes
- Look for structural changes in chromosomes

Lymph Nodes: Components of the lymphatic system, occasionally called "lymph glands." Lymph nodes act as filters, with an internal honeycomb of connective tissue filled with lymphocytes that collect and destroy bacteria and viruses. When the body is fighting an infection, lymphocytes multiply rapidly and produce a characteristic swelling of the lymph nodes.

Liver: A large reddish-brown, glandular vertebrae organ located in the upper-right portion of the abdominal cavity that secretes bile and is active in the formation of certain blood proteins and in the metabolism of carbohydrates, fats, and proteins.

Malignant: Describes a cancerous growth that possesses the ability to invade adjacent tissues and spread distantly to other organs.

Melatonin: Hormone secreted into the bloodstream by the pineal gland.

Meditation: The art of uniting with your Creator to find inner peace and spiritual balance of mind and body.

Metastasize: Refers to cancer that spreads in tissues and organs of the body destructively.

Micronutrient: A substance needed only in small amounts for normal body function.

Minerals: Natural compounds formed through geological processes. Minerals range in composition from pure elements and simple salts to very complex silicates with thousands of known forms.

Microorganism: An organism that is microscopic (too small to be visible to the naked eye). Microorganisms are often described as single-celled, or unicellular, organisms; however, some unicellular protests are visible to the naked eye, and some multicellular species are microscopic. The study of microorganisms is called microbiology.

Necrosis: Death of one or more cells, or a portion of a tissue or organ.

Nutrition: The study of the relationship between diet and the states of health and disease.

Organs: A group of tissues that perform a specific function or group of functions. Usually there is a main tissue and sporadic tissues. The main tissue is unique for the specific organ. For example, the main tissue in the heart is the myocardium, while sporadic tissues are the nervous, blood, connective, etc.

Oxygen: A chemical element with the chemical symbol O and atomic number 8. On earth, it is usually covalently or ionically bonded to other elements.

Pancreas: An organ that manufactures various enzymes for digestion and releases hormones to help control the body's use of carbohydrates. It releases insulin to help each cell absorb glucose to burn as energy. In this way, insulin controls the amount of sugar (glucose) in the blood. Proper pancreatic function is very important to good health.

Phytochemicals: The substances that occur naturally in plants and have been shown in research to possibly prevent or cure disease.

Prostate: An exocrine gland of the male mammalian reproductive system. Its main function is to store and secrete a clear, slightly basic fluid that constitutes up to one-third of the volume of semen.

Prostatectomy: The removal of the prostate gland.

Progesterone: A C-21 steroid hormone involved in the female menstrual cycle, pregnancy, and embryogenesis of humans and other species. Progesterone belongs to a class of hormones called progestogens and is the major naturally occurring human progestogen.

Protein: Compounds composed of hydrogen, oxygen, and nitrogen present in the body and in foods that form complex combinations of amino acids. Proteins are essential for life and are used for growth and repair.

Radiation Therapy: The use of high-energy rays to kill cancer cells. Radiation therapy is local therapy—it affects cancer cells only in the treated area. External radiation does not cause the body to become radioactive.

Selenium: An essential element involved primarily in enzymes that are antioxidants.

Stagin: A method used by physicians to gauge the size and location of a tumor by using information gathered from imaging studies such as CT scans and MRIs, and from pathology tests and physical examinations.

Testicles: Egg-shaped sex glands in the scrotum that secrete male hormones such as testosterone and produce sperm.

Testosterone: The principal male hormone that induces and maintains the changes that take place in males at puberty. In men, the testicles continue to produce testosterone throughout life. There is a decline in the production of testosterone as men age.

Tissues: A connection of interconnected cells that perform a similar function within an organism.

Ultrasound: Testing usin sound waves projected into the body to produce an image of internal organs, structures, tumors, etc. In this procedure, a gel is applied to the patient's skin, and a small device that emits ultrasonic pulses is slowly passed over the area. The sonic image produced is viewed on a monitor.

Vegetables: All parts of an herbaceous plant that humans eat whole or in part. Mushrooms are also considered to be vegetables.

Vitamin D: A fat-soluble vitamin essential to one's health. It regulates the amount of calcium and phosphorus in the blood by improving their absorption. It is necessary for normal growth and formation of bones and teeth. For vitamin D only, one mcg translates to forty IU.

X-rays (X-ray): High-energy radiation used to take pictures of areas inside the body.

Bibliography

ABCs of Prostate Cancer
Joseph E. Oesterling MD
Mark A. Moyad MPH

Advanced Nutrition and Human Metabolism
James L. Goff
Sareen S. Gropper

"A Gift of Health for Dad: Prostate Cancer"
Robin Wallace
Fox NEWS
Web MD Health

American Cancer Society
http://www.cancer.org/dorroot/home/index.asp

American Family Physician
Prostate Cancer Screening
http://www.aafp.org/afp/980800ap/lefevre.html

American Institute for Cancer Research
http://www.aicr.org/site/PageServer

American Journal of Physiology
Endocrinology and Metabolism
http://aipendo.physology.org

American Nutraceutical Association
http://www.ana-jana.org/herbs.cfm

American Prostate Society
www.Ameripros.Org/bph.html

A Primer on Prostate
Donna Pogliano
Phoenix 5 Infro Link Site Cancer
http://www.phoenix5.org/Basics/DPprimer0918.html

The Antioxidant Miracle
Lester Packer PhD
Carol Colman

British Journal of Radiology (BJR)
http://bjr.birjournals.org/

Cancer
Cellular health series
Matthias Rath, MD

Cancer Therapy
Malin Dollinger MD
Margaret Tempero MD

CancerHelp UK
www.cancerhelp.org.uk

Center for Disease Control and prevention
http://www.cdc.gov/index.htm

Centers for Disease Control and Prevention
Nutrition Topics
http://www.gov/nccdphp/dnpa/nutrition/index.htm

The Centre for Unhindered Living
Le Magazine Aug 2001 Report
An Innovative Approach to Cancer
http://www.sciencedirect.com/science

Colman Vernon
http://www.vernoncoleman.com
The Chemistry of Life
Steven Rose

Complete Guide to Prostate Cancer
David G. Bostwick MD, MBA
David Crawford MD
Celestia S. Hizano MD
Mack Roach MD

"Creating Health"
Ageless Body, Timeless Mind
Deepak Chopra MD

Diet and Prostate Cancer
Http://www.patienthealthinternational.com

Diet Nutrition and Prostate Cancer
American Institute for Cancer Research

Dr Joseph Mercola Health Program
http://www.mercola.com

E. Medicine Prostate Cancer
Nutrition Article
Stanley A. Brosman MD

Empty Harvest
Dr. Bernard Jensen
Mark Anderson

Encyclopedia of Natural Medicine
Michael Murray ND
Joseph Pizzorno ND

ENH Evanston North Western Healthcare
http://enh.org/

Experimental Biology and Medicine
http://www.ebmonline.org/

Food Alone Is Not Enough
David W. Rowland

Food Choices for Health
http://www.pcrm.org/health

Food Mood Body
Gary Null

Glyco Science.com
The Nutrition Science Site

http://www.bostwicklaboratories.com
Grading Prostate Cancer
Phoenix 5 Infro Link Site

Guide for Surviving Prostate Cancer
Dr. Patrick Walsh

Guide to Diet and Detoxification
Dr Bernard Jensen

Harper's Illustrated Biochemistry
Robert K. Granner
Daryl K Granner
Peter A. Mayes
Victor W. Rodwell

HEALING by GOD'S Natural Methods
Al Wolfsen

Healing with Whole Foods
Paul Pitchford

Health and Age (Men's Health Center)
http://healthandage.com

Health News
http://www.patienthealthinternational.com

Health Library
http://www.cnn.com/health/library

Healthy Prostate
Arnold Fox MD
Barry Fox PhD

Heart Spring
http://www.ctos.org
GIST Support International
Nutrition and Cancer

Highlights of NCI's Prevention and Control Programs
Http://cancerweb.ncl.ac.uk/cancernet

The Holy Bible
King James Version

Hormonal Drug Increases Survival in Prostate Cancer
http://medicineworld.org/cancer/lead

http://www.givingvoice.org
http://www.nlm.nih.gov/medlineplus/ne

Journal of the National Cancer Institute
http://jnci.oxfordjournals.org/

Journal Article
http://www.springerlink.com/content/j90228u130527u03/

The Human Body in Health and Disease
Darba Janson Cohen
Dena Lin Wood

Huron Valley Urology Associate
Minimizing Prostate Cancer

The Immune System Handbook
Charlene A. Day
Illustrated by Michael O'Regan

Loma Linda University
Adventist Health Studies
http://www.llu.edu/llu/health/abstracts/abstracts2.html

The Intelligent Patient Guide to Prostate Cancer
S. Larry Goldenberg MD
Ian M. Thampson MD

Mayo Clinic.com
http://www.mayoclinic.com

Medline Plus
http://www.nlm.nih.gov/medlineplus/news

Melissa Kaplan's Biochemical Individuality
Chronic Neuroimmune Disease
http://www.anapsid.org/cndbooks/biochem.html/

Ministry of Healing
Ellen G. White

Molecules of Emotion
Candace B. Pert PhD

MSN
Learning & Research
Human Nutrition
Encarta MSN.Com
http://encarta.msn.com/encyclopedia_761556865_2/Human_Nutrition.html

MMP
http://www.mmphealthcare.com

National Cancer Institute
http://www.cancer.gov/prevention/lifestyle.html

National Standard
http://www.naturalstandard.com/

Natural Prostate Health
http://www.healingtherapies.info/natural_prostate_health.htm

Natural Prostate Health
Roger Mason
http://www.oradix.com/health/rogermasonsresearchchapaperth.shtml

New Hope Medical Centre, Inc.
Scottsdale AZ
http://www.newhomedicalcenter.com/

NIH News
National Institutes of Health
http://www.nih.gov

Nutrition and Cancer
WHO IARC
Dr. E. Riboli

Nutrition and Cancer Anti-Cancer Diet
http://www.nutritionj.com/content

Nutrition.org
Diet and Cancer
www.labDiet.com

Nutritional Biochemistry and Metabolism
Edited by
Maria C. Linder

Nutritional Influences on Illness
Melvyn R. Werbach MD

Nutritional Symphomatology: A Professional Guide
David W. Rowland

Optimum Nutrition and Lifestyle for Fighting Prostate Cancer
http://www.brachytherapy.com/prostate-nutrition.html

Optimum Nutrition for the Mind
http://www.mentathealthproject.com

Our Stolen Future: Impotence Likely After Prostate Cancer
Boston Globe
18 January 2005
Ann Barnard (*Globe* staff)

The Patient Guide to Prostate Cancer
Marc B. Barnick MD

Prostate Cancer
David G. Boswick MD
Gregory T. Maclennan MD

Phytochemical
Essential Nutrition Information
Alternative Medicine and Health.com
http://alternative-medecine-and-health.com

Positive Health
Nutrition and Cancer
http://www.positivehealth.com

Prevention of Prostate Cancer
http://www.meb.uni-bonn.de/cancernet/305029.html

Prevention and Treatment of Prostate Cancer
Dietary Intervention
Steven K. Clinton MD,

Prostate
Phoenix 5 Infro Link
http:www.phoenix5.com

The Prostate Book:
Sound Advice on Symptoms and Treatment
Stephen N. Rous MD

Prostate and Cancer
Dr. Seldon Marks MD

Prostate Cancer
American Academy of Family Physicians
http://familydoctor.org/

Prostate Cancer
Detection Inc.
Disease of the Prostate

Prostate Cancer
http://www.systemsbiology.org

Prostate Cancer for Dummies
Paul H. Lange MD

Prostate Cancer: Nutrition
http://www.emedicine.com/med/topic3100.htm

Prostate Cancer Prevention
http://www.yourhealthbase.com

Prostate Cancer Prevention
International Health News Database
Prostate Cancer and Lycopene

Prostate Cancer Prevention
Study to Test Selenium and Vitamin E
July 29, 2001
Vanderbilt-Ingram Cancer Centre

Prostate Cancer Protection Plan
Dr Bob Arnot

Prostate Cancer Special
Foreword by Jadd Moul, MD
Walter Reed Army Medical Center

Prostate Cancer Treatment
ABC News Centre
http://abcnews.go.com/health

Prostate Cancer Treatment Information
http://www.cancerlinksusa.com

Prostate Message and Health
Sunlight and Prostate Cancer
http://www.prostate-massage-and-health.com

Prostate Surgery
Lena Jamnick RN
Robert Nam MD

Prostate Tales:Man's Experiences with Prostate Cancer
Ross Gary
Executive Director Cancer Network

Rayburne W. Goen MD, FACP, FACC
Open Letter
6803 So. Delaware Ave. Tulsa
Oklahoma 74136

Sugars That Heal: The New Healing Science of Glyconutrients
Emil I. Mondoa MD
Mindy Kitel

The Supersystem
Michael Arnoff MD
Indiana University

Thinking through the Body
The Autonomic Nervous System
http://www.thinkbody.com

Transurethral Microwave Thermotherapy of the Prostate
http://www.emedicine.com

MMP
http://www.mmphealthcare.com

Vernon Coleman
Prostate Cancer
www.vernoncoleman.com

Vitamin Research Products
Ward Dean, MD

What are Medications for Incontinence?
http://www.adam.com/democontent/articles/000050_13.htm

What Is Cancer? American Cancer Society
http://www.cancer.org/

Young at Any Age
David W. Rowland

Young Again.org
http://www.youngagain.org

Printed in the United States
133143LV00003B/145-498/P